T0276268

SLOW SEASONS

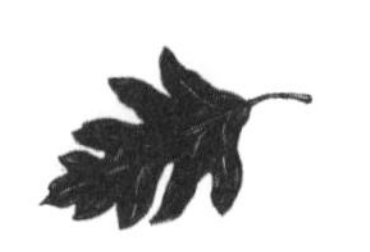

TO NORAH
& ROBERT

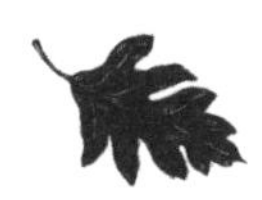

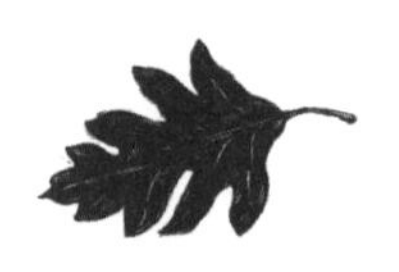

SLOW SEASONS

A Creative Guide to Reconnecting with Nature the Celtic Way

ROSIE STEER

BLOOMSBURY PUBLISHING
LONDON • OXFORD • NEW YORK • NEW DELHI • SYDNEY

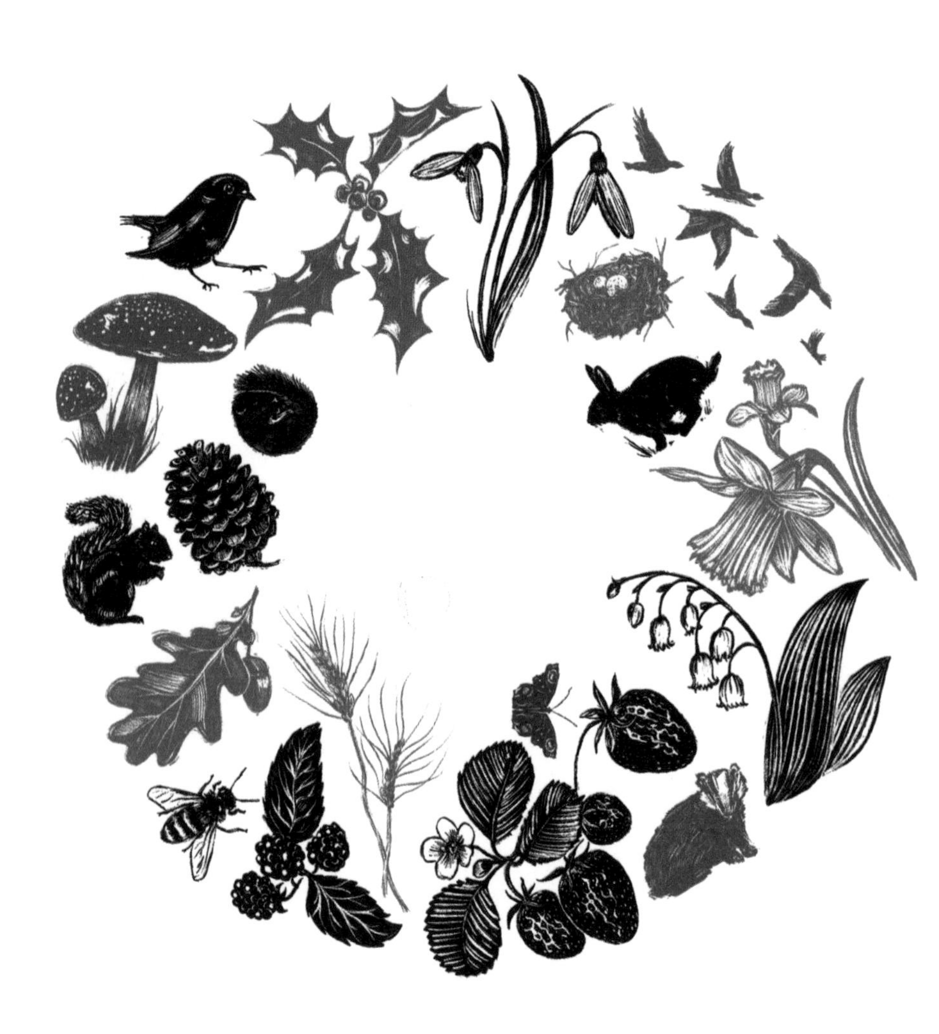

INTRODUCTION

The childish joy of the year's first snowfall. Spotting the first shoots emerge from the earth, a miracle of returning life and energy. The hazy freedom of endless Summer days at the seaside. Inky fingers and the promise of blackberry crumble. The spectacular shedding of Autumn's coat, all tones of russet and gold. The quiet beauty of a frosty Winter day under crystalline blue skies.

The turn of the seasons offers a source of constant wonder in an uncertain world, a reminder of the beauty and small joys that we can find at all times of the year if we slow down and look closely enough. In recent times the healing powers of nature have been more widely recognised, and more of us take our cues from the seasons as an antidote to the sped-up pace of modern life. I'm sure we've all experienced how the natural world can affect our mood – whether from the feeling of Summer abundance, the mood-boosting power of a crisp Autumn day, or, on the flipside, the difficulty getting out of bed in Winter and the relentlessness of stormy, dreich days and perpetually distant springtime.

None of this is new. Our modern understanding of what we now refer to as the Celtic Wheel of the Year echoes the solar events – the solstices and equinoxes – and their rough midpoints, an ancient cycle celebrating the seasons and balance in the natural world. While there is some debate about how old these traditions are and how they came into existence, what is clear is that these cyclical patterns have been passed down over thousands of years. Early Scottish Celts, perhaps like those on the maternal side of my family tree, also believed in a goddess or Earth Mother. In some tales she is depicted as a dual being: as Bride in the warmer months and Cailleach in the colder months. This symbolism has always intrigued me: the idea of Mother Nature as possessing both light and shade, Summer and Winter, her ability to give and to take. I find it comforting, the knowledge that Spring will always arrive eventually, that bad times will come but they will also pass.

Historically, the names of the celebrations in the Celtic Wheel differ depending on whether you follow Anglo-Saxon or Scandinavian traditions or Druid history, and whether you study 1600s' witchcraft or sixties' counterculture in America; but while the dates and names are still contested, there is a shared reverence for the natural world and the cyclical nature of these celebrations, originating from the peaks and troughs of the farming year and the rhythm of the seasons. For simplicity, I have applied the most modern, Scottish interpretations of the names for these ancient festivals to structure my book as it leads you through the year.

There is no one Celtic tradition, no one Scotland, and therefore no one, definitive, set of customs. My influences are from the south of Scotland and its historically contested borders, where my mum was raised in Carlisle just ten miles south of the border, and from where I was born and raised, in Fife in the east of Scotland. This book includes my family's traditions – ones that have been passed down through generations of strong women with busy minds for whom the act of making has had a strong yet unspoken therapeutic effect. Many of these projects I learnt at Mum's kitchen table over Scotch pancakes and jam. Now I make them at my own second-hand kitchen table that has seen everything from candle making to lockdown learning and has the scratches and stains to tell the tales.

SLOW SEASONS IS A CELEBRATION OF THE NOSTALGIC AND THE HOMESPUN; SIMPLE PLEASURES INSPIRED BY THE SEASONS, THAT EVERYONE CAN ENJOY.

The year is marked out by celebrations and instincts deep in my bones: a subconscious part of my upbringing and inheritance I had never questioned, the things we made and did together echoing the seasonal shifts. The rhythm of my life was part of the greater rhythm of my ancestors' traditions and the light and darkness that marked their lives. A wheel that kept on turning.

It was when I was noting down my monthly, seasonal to-do lists that I started to join the dots between my heritage and the comforting rituals that I had made for myself. The things I made and celebrated not only kept my hands busy, stilling my whirring brain and helping me to slow down, but also made me feel more connected to the traditions of the past, reviving them for the present.

Since childhood I had quietly struggled with my anxieties beneath a successful surface, but I was in the no-man's land of my mid-twenties when the intrusive thoughts of OCD (Obsessive Compulsive Disorder) took over, trapping me in patterns of unhealthy behaviour. The reality of the working world, complexities of relationships, and relentlessness of day-to-day life and passage of time intensified my symptoms. I was lost and felt utterly alone and unspeakably low. I could get myself to work and function well as friendly teacher Miss Steer, but every night I would have to go straight home to bed, as Rosie was plagued by constant migraines, unstoppable tears and suicidal thoughts. Feeling so lost, I was looking for other ways – any way – to feel a little more connected and less at sea.

In the end, it was the small things I held onto. Even my beloved books – English graduate and newly qualified teacher that I then was – betrayed me, unable to focus on the words as they swam in my brain. Audiobooks offered something of a solace. So did the seasons. In particular, the depiction of the farming year in *Sunset Song*, written by Lewis Grassic Gibbon, captured my imagination, where the transience of the seasons was not a source of anxiety but part of the cycle of nature and its reliable progression. This made me realise how connected we humans are with this wider cycle and made me feel less alone. I eased back into reading with stories about Scottish traditions, folk and fairy stories, ancient flower symbolism, rituals and recipes. It offered me a lifeline and a language through which to explore my roots. The more I learnt, the more I began to realise that this gave an official name and history to some of the traditions I too celebrated when growing up.

We always marked the passing of the seasons in our household. Ostara came with Granda tending Spring bulbs and Gran decorating eggs. In St Andrews, we ran into the North Sea for one very cold 'tradition' to mark the arrival of Beltane. We spent the endless days of Litha outdoors, usually on bike rides along the Fife coastal path with a flask of something and homemade treats as fuel. We celebrated Samhain by carving neeps and eating simple suppers, and saw in Yule with candles and evergreens decorating the house.

Unwittingly, by revisiting these rituals I was beginning to practise mindfulness and slow living, lifelines that would eventually avert my panic attacks on the way to work and carve out pockets of quiet contentment. With time, a cocktail of anti-depressants and anxiety medications, failed therapy sessions, a long waiting list and the eventual, life-changing wisdom of my NHS therapist Ronnie, and support of my partner Al and my family, I began to find my way back to myself.

Even at my lowest ebb, small celebrations, routines and wee joys such as collecting conkers or arranging a posy of wildflowers, offered me purpose. They triggered a nostalgia that took me all the way back to childhood: from walks on our local beach collecting pebbles to curating the nature table. A quiet childhood that was simple – old-fashioned, maybe – and all the more comforting for it. I started to document my love of nature and old ways, seeking a community of like-minded souls online. I started to realise that other people were listening to my seasonal stories and responding with their own. Slowly, the fog that had clouded my mind for so long started to dissipate.

In an uncertain world there was comfort in the twin forces of nature and nostalgia. Our patterns of thinking are the well-trodden path: familiar, safe, quick and easy. For me this was a sped-up pace of living that played a role in my mental illness: you just had to look at the shops' Easter egg displays in January to feel like time was passing so quickly, leaving you always behind.

Modern living felt like constantly hurtling towards the next holiday, speeding up the seasonal cycle, making us ever wanting. In many ways I find that this sped-up way of living and consuming that is fed to us reflects how the world tries to make us live our lives, a pressure I felt keenly as an insecure achiever, conscious that everyone else was moving on to the next achievement, the next 'milestone' ticked off the life list while I was left behind – living alone and working a high-stress job I had fallen out of love with. It's no wonder we never seem fully satisfied and are left feeling burnt out.

Maybe it's because the world is so complex and busy that we cling to goals and achievements to carve out a sense of control, to shape our own narratives. But maybe there's another way we can be? Forging a new path in the forest of life takes time and effort. You need to muster your commitment to new patterns of thinking, exposing yourself to new experiences – and yes, sometimes the attendant anxieties they bring – to create a healthier path that, over time, will become well-trodden.

> I KNOW NOW THERE IS A WAY THAT WE CAN SLOW DOWN AND TUNE INTO NATURE'S RHYTHMS TO GET BACK TO WHAT'S IMPORTANT – TO GET BACK TO OURSELVES.

I knew something had to change for me, and it turned out my new path was actually a very old one.

I'd always felt connected with nature until the disconnect of my depression took its roots in my mind, then I began to notice it anew, all over again. At the same time, I started to realise how connecting with the seasons and the very acts of nurturing, making and celebrating the small things had helped heal me all along – often without me even noticing. This is why I wanted to, had to, write this book. To help others find something to celebrate in all seasons of life: to find light and shade, to find balance.

Despite what society tells us, I strongly believe that a life lived fully is a life lived in the smaller moments. In *Slow Seasons* I want to highlight the Celts' sense of seasonal balance, an understanding that there might be times of darkness but that light will come – and, what's more, there is always light to be found within those dark times. Our ancestors had it right: time to sow, time to grow, time to harvest and time to rest. The Celtic Wheel of the Year is as much about a mindset as it is a practice: the seasons are fluid, ever-changing and evolving, and we are too. The way to capture the moment is to slow down and look within, to simplify and celebrate the everyday. I'll pop the kettle on – you pull up a chair.

IMB

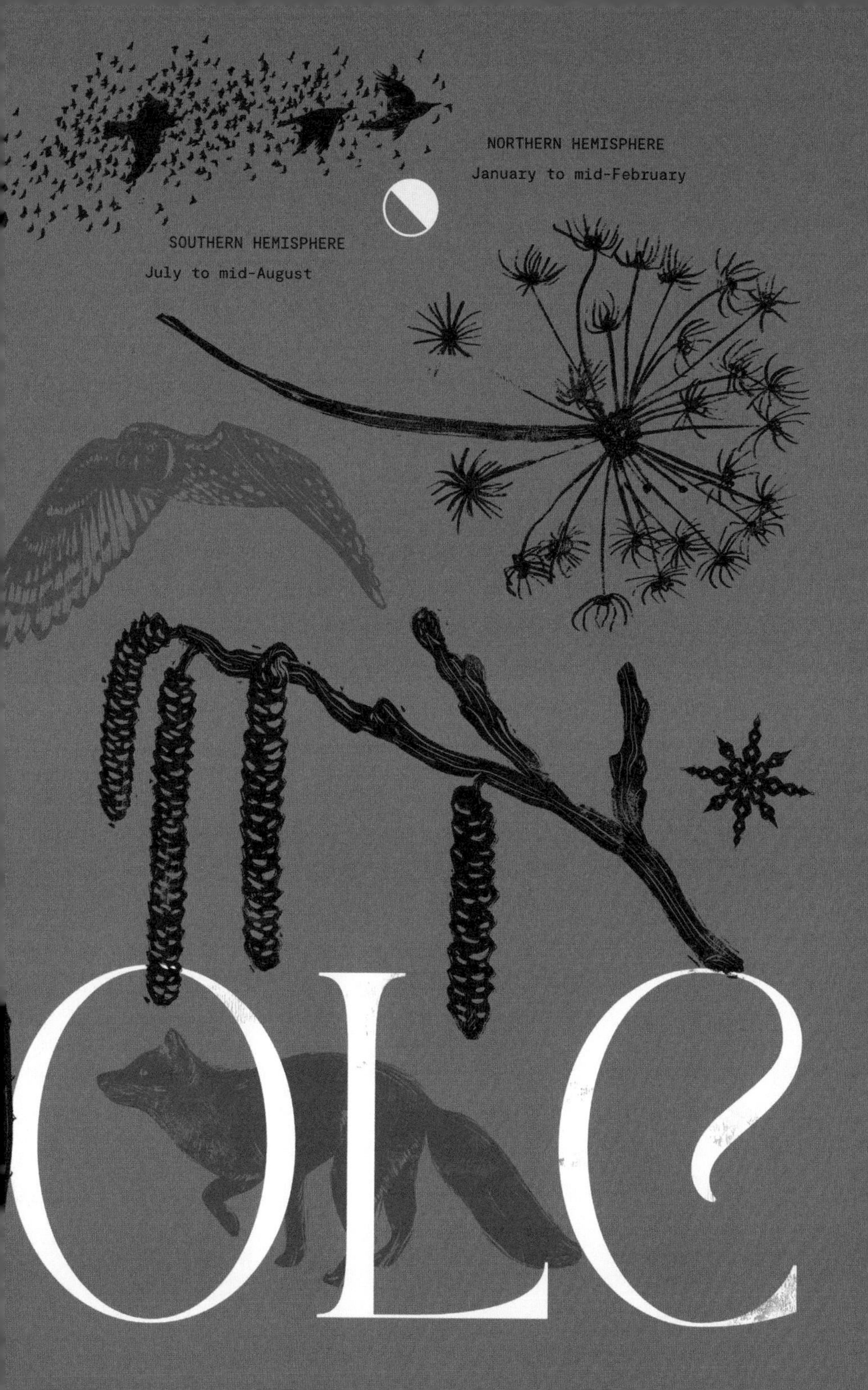
NORTHERN HEMISPHERE
January to mid-February
SOUTHERN HEMISPHERE
July to mid-August

REFLECTING & HIBERNATING

The contrast between the sparkle of Christmas and the greyness of January, alongside the narrative of self-improvement, busyness and denial of the post-festive period meant that I used to intensely dislike the start of the year.

However, there is another way of looking at this blank slate. There is quiet potential in this time: its opportunity and whispered promise, our powerlessness in the face of nature. There is hope in it all – the regenerative power of the new year.

Taking their cues from nature, our Celtic ancestors long associated this period with hunkering down, rest and regeneration. They savoured the slowness of Winter. Something about this annual rhythm of slowing down and letting go resonates deeply within us; indeed, evidence has recently been discovered that early humans would hibernate to survive harsh glacial Winters.

And yet, in our modern world with all its stimulation and the value society attaches to the new and the shiny, it can become all too tempting to rush towards Spring and the life, colour and activity it symbolises – particularly as the first Easter eggs tend to appear in shops around now. However, speeding towards the next season can leave us feeling burnt out as we battle low light levels, which promote the production of the hormone melatonin that makes us want to sleep more, and our brains encourage us to slow, to rest and to nurture our bodies.

What's more, this contemporary narrative denies us the crucial joy of living in the here and now. So much life can be found in the midst of Winter, from the impossibly green shoots of the first snowdrops – a miracle beneath a brown carpet of bracken – to the song of a robin perched on a bare branch, chest puffed up in pride: small daily miracles of resilience and hope.

For many of us, the pace of the world makes it challenging to slow down and allow our bodies and minds time to become accustomed to the colder months. Electricity, lighting and central heating are all modern conveniences that make our Winters easier to survive, of course – but they also mask our inner signals to slow, rest and revive. I'm certain this is why many of us are left feeling low in the Winter months: the world keeps turning and we are expected to carry on at the same pace, lest we be left behind.

Looking to our ancestors can provide a compromise. Since I started following the Celtic Wheel, I've been much more attuned to the in-between seasons marked by the Celts that not only celebrate the magic of the moment but signal a movement forwards. Imbolc (pronounced 'IMM-bolk'), the festival of fire and light, is the Celtic feast celebrating the very beginning of Spring – a pivotal moment of change that signifies new beginnings, growth and renewal. We are still in Winter, but look closely and you'll notice the seasons beginning to shift little by little, day by day as the light grows stronger, little by little, day by day.

Imbolc always reminds me of Granda, who loved to garden and – like me – hated being trapped indoors over Winter. On visits to my grandparents' house, I would join him, wrapped up in many, many layers, and watch him tend seedlings in his greenhouse. When I was older, he would encourage my windowsill garden efforts from afar, sharing tips for tending fruit and vegetables at home. Making the most of the present season isn't always easy, particularly in Winter, but a subtle shift in thinking can help us be more mindful: sowing seeds indoors; getting outside, whatever the weather; gently planning for longer and lighter days.

> FOR ME, CARVING OUT SMALL RITUALS EVERY DAY HAS BECOME MY WAY TO RECLAIM THE LIGHT AND CHANGE THE NARRATIVE OF BUSYNESS.

Lighting a candle over breakfast; slipping back beneath the sheets with a hot cup of tea in my favourite mug before a busy day; spotting the first snowdrops on my walk to work; making something with my hands at the weekend and losing myself in the craft. These are all wee moments that centre me, bring me back to the here and now and give light at a time it is in short supply.

It's even more vital than ever to show yourself kindness at this dark time. I hope to give you a few ideas for how to do just that in this chapter. Savour the slowness of Winter: start to note the small changes around you as the Earth begins to turn back towards the sun and the days get just that wee bit longer. But don't rush time: beauty can be found in the brown and grey and white of Winter.

Seasonal Celebrations at Home

In the Celtic Wheel of the Year, Imbolc marks the halfway point between the Winter Solstice, Yule, and the Spring Equinox, Ostara. This quiet period should be one of rest and regeneration, not impossible resolutions and self-flagellation. Reflecting compassionately on the past year and quietly planning for what's to come is a kinder way to start the year. When it's cold and miserable outdoors, I love nothing more than making the house as cosy as possible. With candles, blankets and comfy loungewear, it becomes a nest that I have little desire to leave. My fairy lights don't go away until at least Ostara – if at all. Whatever your Winter haven looks like, embrace it a little longer.

Gentle Reflection

If, like me, you find this time difficult, our priorities should, rightfully, include resting and mentally surviving the Winter months. However, if you feel drawn to the fresh slate of the new year, then ensure your reflection comes from a place of kindness. I don't believe in impossible resolutions or over-ambitious goals, but rather looking back on the past season with care and setting smaller aims. While some feel the fresh impetus of the new year in January, I tend to do this at the start of the school year (it's the teacher in me), and others do it in Spring. That intrinsic motivation, by definition, must come from within, so engage in these activities whenever the energy does arrive (but don't beat yourself up if it doesn't) and speak to yourself as you would a friend and do what works for you. I don't get on well with resolutions and I don't like to slip into ruminating and regret, so instead I look back on photos and journal notes for meaningful moments from the year passed, using them as inspiration for some small goals. Which moments and feelings do I want to recreate this year? What am I most grateful for? Where would I like to be this time next year? (Literally, emotionally.) I am a big believer in the power of writing things down: noting some key words or even making a mood board helps to keep my focus positive rather than punitive. I tend to keep this to myself rather than sharing – but if you want a friend to hold you to account and keep you on track, then choose someone who is going to motivate in a way that works for you.

Planning with Kindness

When I was on the waiting list for some intense and long-needed therapy, a doctor once 'prescribed' this to me: 'Just plan something to look forward to!' At the time, I felt completely dismissed – I felt like nobody believed I was sick – but post-therapy, I can see that she had the right idea, she just went about it clumsily (at best). Fixing moments in the diary – no matter how big or small – does give you a sense of forward momentum and purpose. This period is an ideal time to plan some simple things to look forward to. Perhaps plan a short break, or even a day trip close to home – visits abroad aren't always possible or affordable, but making a holiday-at-home weekend can be just as fun, and doesn't need to be restricted to Summer. I find that researching beforehand makes me look forward to it all the more; it could be a trip centred around visiting a destination bakery, a stately home or some natural wonder, just because. I plan a mini-itinerary with a list of places to go, things to see and do and, most importantly, food to eat – again, I can't help my inner teacher! But if you prefer to be more spontaneous, then explore to your heart's content. A one-off trip, even if just for a day, can feel like a holiday, all for the cost of a train ticket. I find such days vital for topping up my inspiration levels.

Nature Tonic

On days when the wind whistles down the chimney or the rain pelts the pavements, going for a walk might be your last priority. However, wrapping up and doing just that can be a surprising tonic. Choose your location and set a time limit – maybe a loop through your favourite woods with the promise of a hot bath when you get home, or an invigorating walk along the promenade that ends at your favourite café. The thought of a reward always helps – and if food-based, it tastes all the sweeter. On a serious note though, I always feel better for the fresh air even if I almost constantly complain; nature puts my worries into vital perspective and exposure to the elements definitely makes me appreciate my cosy home more. Bring a flask of something warm with you and dress for the weather: thermals and wellies are your friends. If the weather really is that terrible, then reading about nature and looking at images of nature have been found to provide similar benefits. Over lockdown I found just watching the silver birch over the road, swaying in the breeze, brought me enormous comfort, as did noticing its first buds and spotting its resident avian visitors. When a properly cold, crisp, frosty day comes along, I fall in love with Winter all over again – looking out at the glittering rooftops, seeing the pale pink and lilac skies of a frosty sunrise, and feeling the crunch of icy leaves and branches beneath my feet all make me feel alive.

Homemade Fat Balls for Birds

If you have a garden or even just a windowsill, it's a lovely idea to set up a bird feeder now that food is becoming scarcer. As well as helping local wildlife, this craft has the bonus of welcoming birds into your environment where you can observe them up close – an impressive Winter sight. To make homemade bird seed fat balls, mix peanut butter with a little plain flour or rolled oats blitzed in a blender, shape into balls with your hands and then roll in generous amounts of mixed seeds suitable for birds. Or get crafty and cover natural objects such as pine cones, acorns or seed heads with a thin layer of peanut butter and then a generous coating of seeds before hanging them from branches with twine. Make sure you go for all-natural peanut butter low in salt and without additives such as palm oil – the main ingredient should be peanuts. It's great for smaller birds that can struggle to access and open whole nuts in bird feeders, giving them an easily digestible source of protein and fat.

Celebrating Imbolc

Imbolc is a celebration of returning light, growth and fertility that takes place on 1 or 2 February. It coincides with the Christian holiday of Candlemas and both celebrations are associated with light and hope. Fire symbolises both purification and protection, welcoming the return of the sunlight, while candles are frequently lit to symbolise renewal. In Scottish tradition, the hearth fire was usually extinguished and re-lit, with candles in each room and a broom placed by the door to symbolise the cleaning out of the old and celebration of the new. It is so comforting to me to know that the coming of Spring has been celebrated for thousands of years. It makes me feel quite emotional and certainly helps to put things into perspective – a reminder of the cycle of the seasons and the timeless certainty they can provide in our tumultuous modern world. I always light the stove for Imbolc, to echo my ancestors' tradition, and light more candles than is strictly necessary as I set the table (see page 22 for how to make your own candles). A wintry candlelit movie night, nestled in cushions and throws and eating a bowl of fresh, homemade popcorn is my dream cosy night in. I like making plain popping corn (buy a supermarket packet and pop according to the instructions), then sprinkling it with a little ground cinnamon, orange zest, soft brown sugar and sea salt.

CANDLE MAKING

Candles have long been associated with Imbolc or St Brigid's Day and Candlemas, during which church candles are blessed for the coming year. Even in pre-Christian times, Imbolc (Imbolg in Irish Gaelic) was associated with goddess Brigid who was honoured at the beginning of February with fire and feasting.

Candles have been used for thousands of years. First made by the Romans, with papyrus wicks dipped in animal fat, they were used both practically and spiritually, having a long association with religious ceremonies. Candles were mainly made from foul-smelling, smoky tallow until the Middle Ages when beeswax candles became popular in churches and wealthy homes. More affordable spermaceti and paraffin waxes came next, until the invention of the light bulb.

These days we know that paraffin, the main ingredient in most high-street candles, can cause great harm to the planet and to our bodies. Choosing a natural wax is a matter of personal preference, but the likes of soy and beeswax are much better as natural, renewable resources. Beeswax, a by-product of honey making, burns up to five times as long as paraffin, with a bright light, and it is a natural 'ioniser' – removing dirt and pollen from the air. Soy wax also has a longer burn-time than paraffin and is vegan. I favour it for making scented candles, as it can take on other scents and is less expensive.

Making your own candles is a deeply comforting sensory experience during the dull, dark Winter months and encourages slowness and focus: the soft feel of the wax beneath your fingertips; the intoxicating scent as you slowly stir the wax; the golden, flickering light as your candles burn and glow. They are surprisingly simple to make, and immensely satisfying.

I like to use everyday objects for my candles, such as recycled jam jars or thrifted enamel mugs. Those I have gifted candles to often return their containers – a thrifty, if not-so-subtle, hint! A little initial outlay on wicks, wax and fragrances is worth the investment to make and gift your own candles for a fraction of the price of those on the high street.

TIPS

- You don't need any specialist equipment – unless you plan to go into production! I use an old pan and an old, chipped glass jug dedicated to candle making, plus a thermometer that had seen better days.
- Beeswax pellets are easier to use but more expensive – ask your local honey seller if they can get you bars of wax, which you can cut into small chunks.
- You might notice a small dip on the surface of your candle, which is caused by temperature sensitivity. You can remedy this by topping up with more wax once the candle has set. Or for a professional finish: invest in a thermometer to make sure the mixture reaches pouring point; warm the candle receptacle in a low oven to avoid rapid temperature changes; and leave your candle to set in a room that is neither too hot nor too cold.
- Never leave a burning candle unattended.
- Always trim your wick to no more than 5mm before burning to prevent the candle from smoking and leaving black stains on the receptacle – or even on your wall.
- So the scent can be best enjoyed, place your candle away from draughts, preferably at nose height in the middle of the room.
- Always burn your candle for long enough that the wax melts all the way across the surface to prolong its life, otherwise the candle will start to 'tunnel' and you will be left with excess, unburnt wax.
- Invest in a candle snuffer to avoid blowing hot wax all over your surfaces. I learnt this the hard way! I found mine at a vintage fair.
- If you do spill wax on a surface, always wait for it to dry and set so it is easier to scrape off.
- If you spill wax on fabric, it might pop off with the back of a spoon or palette knife when set; if it doesn't, place a piece of kitchen paper under and on top of the waxy mark, place a tea towel on top and iron through the towel – the heat should melt the wax onto the absorbent surface of the kitchen paper. If the wax was coloured you may need to use a stain remover. Wash as usual.

HAND POURED CANDLE

You'll need a prepared wick – you can find these cheaply online or make you own. When choosing oils, ensure they are suitable for candle making, otherwise they could be flammable and cause injuries. If making the candle with beeswax, leave it unscented – the honey scent alone is special enough.

YOU WILL NEED

- Old cloth or newspaper
- Heatproof jar or container (candle receptacle)
- Electronic weighing scales
- Soy wax flakes or beeswax pellets (see tips)
- Candle fragrance oil or essential oils (optional – see above)
- Large, heatproof jug
- Small jug
- Pre-waxed wick
- A large pan
- Palette knife (for stirring)
- Culinary thermometer
- Flameproof mat
- Sharp pair of scissors

Cover a work surface with newspaper or an old cloth to catch drips, then lay out your materials and equipment so that everything is to hand.

Measure everything out: fill the jar or receptacle in which you wish to make your candle with water up to the height you want for your candle. Weigh the water, note the number in grams, then empty out the container and thoroughly dry.

Wax takes up more space than water, so to work out how much you need, multiply the water weight by 0.8. To work out how much fragrance oil you need, multiply the wax weight by 0.08 (I use 8% of candle fragrance oil for a nice, strong scent).

Weigh the corresponding amount of soy wax flakes or beeswax into the large jug and set aside. Weigh the fragrance oil, if using, into the small jug and set aside, too.

Prepare the candle receptacle by sticking your wick to the base, pressing it firmly into the middle.

Fill the pan with a few centimetres of water and place the jug of wax in the pan. Place the pan over a medium heat and bring the water to a gentle simmer. Make sure that the water doesn't evaporate, or the bottom of the jug can scorch.

Stir the wax regularly, using the palette knife, until it starts to turn into a pale yellow liquid. At this point, insert the thermometer into the wax and keep your eye on the temperature.

If using soy wax, continue to heat until it reaches 65°C, or until the wax has all melted and is completely clear. For a beeswax candle, heat the wax to around 70°C.

Turn off the heat and carefully remove the jug from the pan, using oven gloves to protect your hands (watch the bottom for drips). If using beeswax, skip to the next step. If making a scented soy candle, place the jug on a heatproof mat and slowly pour in the fragrance oil. Stir slowly and continually for at least 2 minutes to ensure the fragrance is evenly distributed through the wax.

Now you're ready to pour your candle: slowly and steadily pour the wax from the jug into the prepared candle receptacle. The wick will fall to one side, so either hold it until the wax starts to set (this should happen quite quickly) or use your stirring knife to prop it up.

Leave the candle to set: it will turn from a yellowy liquid to white solid. Even if it looks set, don't move it for a good few hours as it may still be liquid inside.

For best results, set the candle aside to cure for at least a week before burning. When you're ready to use (or gift) the candle, trim the wick to 5mm with a sharp pair of scissors.

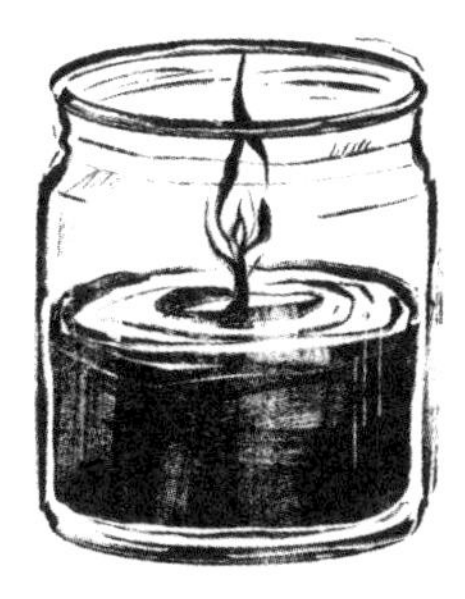

ENVELOPE CUSHION COVER

This all-in-one or envelope cushion cover is simple to make so is great for beginners, as you can make something beautiful and functional in under an hour. Once you've learnt this method, making your own cushion covers is an easy and lovely way to update your décor through the seasons. This craft is perfect for hunkering down at home on a wintry afternoon.

YOU WILL NEED

- 1 square cushion pad (you can buy these from a haberdashery or just reuse a cushion insert you already have) – the standard size is 45 × 45cm
- Measuring tape
- Fabric, washed and pressed – see method for dimensions
- Tailor's chalk or a pen
- Ruler
- Scissors
- Iron and ironing board
- Pins
- Sewing machine
- Thread that matches the fabric

To work out the fabric dimensions, measure the cushion pad with the measuring tape. For the width, add a 2cm seam allowance; and for the length, double the width (including seam allowance) and add 10cm to allow for the envelope to overlap and hide the cushion pad – so for a 45cm cushion pad, your measurements would be 47 × 104cm.

Transfer your measurements to the fabric using tailor's chalk or a pen and a ruler and cut out the fabric. (Or you could give a haberdasher your measurements and they can do this for you.)

Take the short end of your fabric and create a double hem (this will be the edge of your envelope opening): fold the fabric over 1cm, 'wrong' sides (the underside of the pattern) together, press with the iron, then fold the fabric over again by another 1cm. Press, then pin into place.

Set your sewing machine to straight stitch and sew the hem, remembering to finish your stitches at the start and end by using the backstitch function for a couple of stitches.

Repeat to create a double hem for the other short end of fabric.

Now that you've hemmed the opening, you're ready to assemble the cushion: place the fabric right side up on your ironing board. Bring the hemmed ends in towards each other, overlapping them by 10cm – this will be the opening of the envelope. Press then pin the unsewn edges together.

Straight stitch the two unsewn sides of the cushion 1cm in from the edge.

Trim the corners down to 5mm to remove excess fabric, then turn the cushion (which is currently inside out) so that it is right sides out. If you struggle to get the corners into neat points, use your scissors to push them out (but be careful they don't go through).

Give the cushion cover another press, then insert the cushion pad.

Seasonal Celebrations of Nature

The period in the lead-up to Imbolc is one of quietness, reminding us of the power of rest and retreat. In deep Winter, nature slows but it doesn't stop. If you look carefully, so much beauty can be found in the wild, dark season, as can hints of the Spring that will soon follow. Imbolc reminds us of the power of transformation after withdrawing and surrendering to Winter. It is a crucial moment of balance, of finding hope and resilience at the bleakest seeming times.

At first glance outside, everything seems bare and stark. However, if you look closely you will be able to spot the first, wee hints of Spring to come soon. I always look for catkins – long, thin clusters of tiny flowers that trees use to reproduce – as a first sign of Spring stirring. Hazel and alder catkins can be seen by rivers and streams, while pussy willow, with its mink-coloured fluffy catkins, can be found in florists.

Even though the world still seems so cold, the first shoots and buds appear in the lead-up to Imbolc – most notably the first snowdrops of the year, which are everyone's favourite herald of Spring. Galanthophiles – snowdrop fans – gather to celebrate at festivals up and down the UK. And it's easy to see the obsession: the fragile, drooping flowers seem delicate and they are a timely reminder that Spring will be on its way soon.

Due to scarce food supplies in Winter, animals can be more inquisitive around humans, so keep a look out for them in gardens and green spaces, as foxes enter their breeding season around this time; if you don't see them, you might still hear their ear-piercing scream. Deer are a common sight in the countryside, particularly at dawn and dusk, seen through the bare branches – they were frequent and adorable visitors to my parents' garden in the country, growing bolder during the colder days.

As the weather warms, queen bees emerge from hibernation to find a place to build their nests. Ladybirds also appear as the Earth begins to tilt closer to the sun. Insects find early nectar in crocuses, one of the first Spring flowers to bloom.

At dusk, keep your eyes peeled for flocks of starlings swirling overhead. Birds of prey also start to swoop over woodlands and countryside on clear days, asserting their territories. Growing birdsong can also be heard from common blackbirds and thrushes.

Look out for Winter wildfowl such as mallards and tufted ducks on lakes and other bodies of freshwater. If you're at the beach, there's still a surprising amount to see in rockpools – marine snails don't hibernate and seaweed grows all year round.

A major perk of the dwindling daylight is surely being awake to see spectacular Winter sunrises and sunsets. In the lead-up to Imbolc, you might start to notice the days lengthening minute by minute – by the end of January there's a whole extra hour of daylight compared with the beginning of the month, which feels like a small but important victory over the darkness.

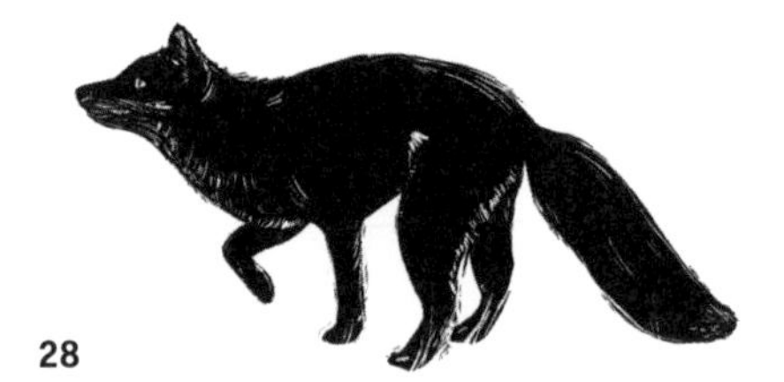

MAKING MARMALADE MEMORIES

Making marmalade is one of my favourite rituals during this dark season. Seville oranges are traditionally used in this preserve, and their brief season coincides with the coldest, darkest days of January, bringing a taste of Mediterranean colour and flavour to the kitchen. I eagerly await their arrival in my local greengrocer, and usually manage to snap them up towards the end of the month. Bigger supermarkets tend to stock them as well, and you can buy them by the kilo.

Preserving is often associated with Summer, but this slow ritual is perfect for Winter weekends. Marmalade is not something to make in haste and tastes all the better for it. Call this culinary mindfulness: each step is a feast for the senses. If you've never made your own marmalade, I urge you to give this a go. Making your own is tastier than anything you can buy in the shops, as you can customise it to your own tastes, including texture (chunky peel or finely shredded) and set (soft and yielding or thick enough to stick to your ribs – the latter is my preference!)

Some historians trace the origins of marmalade to Scotland, though it may seem far removed from exotic Seville orange groves. Marmalade has been linked with the Sutherland Clan, as a notebook from 1683 containing one of the first recorded recipes resides at Dunrobin Castle in the Highlands. Early marmalade was made by pounding the fruit in a pestle and mortar to make a thick mixture similar to quince paste.

The first published Scottish cookery book, *A New and Easy Method of Cookery*, refers to the 'chipped' style preserve in 1752. Modern marmalade as we would recognise it is attributed to the Keiller family, who apparently bought a load of discounted oranges from a cargo ship stuck in Dundee after a storm, and invented marmalade. They went on to create the first marmalade factory in 1797 and popularised the preserve.

MARMALADE

Marmalade making may seem daunting, but the high pectin levels in the fruit mean it's one of the easier preserves to master as the pectin helps with setting. If you break it down into stages you won't go wrong: softening the fruit, extracting the pectin and adding the sugar to make the preserve.

Most recipes use a 1:2 ratio of fruit: sugar. Trust me – this lip-puckering fruit needs it. I love the caramel note that demerara gives my staple marmalade recipe below.

MAKES 6 X 450G JARS

1 kg Seville oranges, washed and scrubbed
2.5 litres water
2 kg demerara sugar

You will need
Muslin, string and a jam thermometer

Place the muslin in a sieve and set over a large, heavy-based pan or preserving pan. Halve the oranges and squeeze their juice into the muslin-lined sieve. Cut each half in half again and pull out the flesh, pips and membrane, into the muslin.

Tie the muslin together tightly with some string to form a bag and place in the pan.

On a chopping board, cut the peel into strips – I like mine nice and thin but whatever size you choose, make sure to cut the peel consistently so that it cooks evenly.

Add the shredded peel to the pan with the water. Place over a medium–high, heat and bring to the boil. Reduce the heat and simmer for 2 hours, or until the peel is cooked through.

Remove the muslin bag and set it aside to cool completely. Wash your jars in warm, soapy water, then transfer them to a low oven (around 100°C) to dry – this will sterilise them and prevent the hot marmalade cracking a cold jar. Boil metal lids in a small pan of boiling water until you are ready to use them. Put a couple of saucers in the fridge or freezer to cool down (depending on how warm your kitchen is).

Once cooled, squeeze the liquid from the muslin bag into the marmalade mixture in the pan. Return to the heat and bring it to a simmer again. Add the sugar. Be careful as the liquid may bubble up considerably at this point. Continue simmering, stirring it regularly, until the sugar is completely dissolved.

Increase the heat and boil rapidly until the marmalade reaches 104°C on a jam thermometer. You can also check the set by placing a teaspoon of the marmalade onto one of the cold saucers. Chill it in the fridge for 1–2 minutes, then put your finger through it: if the surface of the jam wrinkles and your finger leaves a clear line,

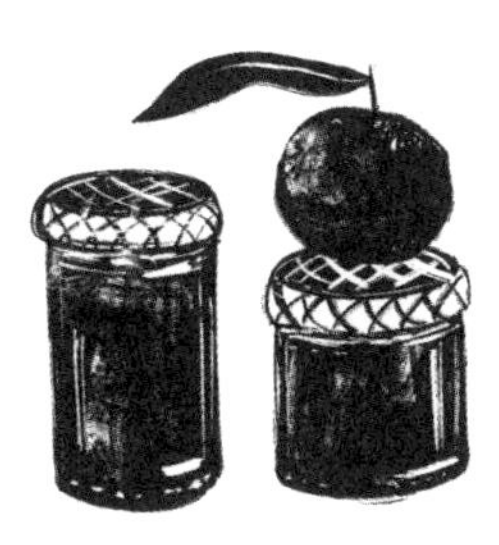

it's ready. If not, return your saucer to the fridge or freezer and continue boiling the marmalade; check again every few minutes.

Once it's ready, turn off the heat and let it sit for 20 minutes or so to let the peel settle. Spoon the marmalade into the warm sterilised jars and carefully put the lids on when everything is still warm.

The marmalade will keep well in a cool, dark place for a couple of years if the jars are properly sterilised. Once the jar is open, store the marmalade in the fridge.

Variations

Blood orange and cardamom marmalade: follow the same steps as above but substitute Seville oranges for blood oranges and an equal amount of sugar rather than double the amount. Stir through half a teaspoon of freshly ground cardamom once the jam has sat and cooled before bottling.

Clementine and vanilla marmalade: follow the same steps as above but substitute the Seville oranges for clementines and an equal amount of sugar rather than double the amount, plus stir through two teaspoons of vanilla extract once the jam has sat and cooled before bottling.

Note: both these variations will have a slightly looser set as the fruit contains less pectin, but you can help it along by adding the juice of a lemon and its rind and pips in the muslin. For both of these variations, you may need to boil the fruit peel for less time than with Seville oranges, but then need to boil for longer after adding the sugar to get the correct set.

MARMALADE BOSTOCKS

A bostock is a French pastry that was invented to use up stale brioche. Stale pastries never seem to be a problem in my house, so I buy sliced brioche to make these bostocks: think of them as a hybrid of a brioche bun and an almond croissant. Marmalade is the perfect foil for sweet brioche, topped with almond frangipane and baked until oozing and golden.

SERVES 5

120g butter
120g caster sugar
1 large free-range egg
Zest of 1 orange
120g ground almonds
5 slices of brioche
75g marmalade
Boiling water (optional)
Flaked almonds, for sprinkling
Icing sugar, for dusting

Pre-heat the oven to 180°C/Fan 160°C/Gas Mark 4. Line a tray with kitchen foil.

In a bowl, beat the butter and sugar until light and fluffy, then add the egg, orange zest and ground almonds to make a firm paste. This is your frangipane.

Spread the brioche slices out on the foil-lined tray.

Warm the marmalade in a bowl in the microwave, adding a little boiling water if you need to loosen it further.

Spread about 1 tablespoon of marmalade on top of each piece of brioche as you would spread toast, then top with 2 tablespoons of frangipane in the middle of each and spread over the top of the marmalade (ensure you cover it all or it will burn).

Add a sprinkling of flaked almonds on top and bake for 15–20 minutes, until golden brown.

Remove from the oven, dust with icing sugar and serve.

Tip

This makes enough frangipane topping for ten bostocks – so either double the amount of brioche slices and marmalade and have a pastry party, or use the frangipane for other recipes or keep leftovers for the next batch of bostocks: it will keep in the fridge for one week or in the freezer for a month. Simply slice a piece of frozen frangipane off the block and top the bostocks, increasing the cooking time by 5 minutes.

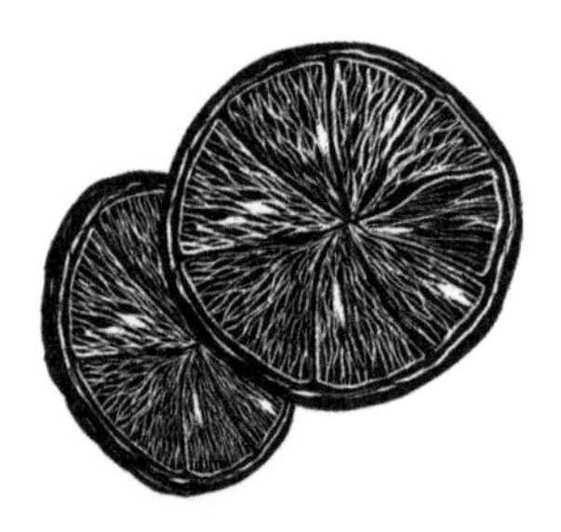

MARMALADE CINNAMON BUNS

Hunkering down and making home a cosy, welcoming Winter haven begins in the kitchen for me – always. Weekdays might be spent on autopilot, but when I have longer windows of time at the weekend, I love to plan a therapeutic baking afternoon – the most precious ingredient in these marmalade cinnamon buns is time. They are best eaten on the day, but can be warmed in the oven the following day, and can be frozen individually (without the marmalade glaze) for up to 1 month. Defrost and warm in the oven, then glaze.

MAKES APPROX. 12

For the dough

40g butter
150ml semi-skimmed milk
7g fast action yeast sachet
250g strong flour
25g caster sugar
Pinch of sea salt
Zest of 1 large orange

For the filling

60g butter
1 tsp ground cinnamon
60g soft brown sugar
75g marmalade

For the glaze

2 tbsp marmalade, loosened with a little boiling water

Place the butter and milk together in a heatproof jug and melt in the microwave, or place in a milk pan over a low heat until melted. Allow the mixture to cool to body temperature.

Mix the yeast into the warm butter and milk and set it aside for about 15 minutes – it will start to froth a little.

Place the flour, caster sugar, salt and orange zest in the bowl of a stand mixer fitted with the dough hook or in a large mixing bowl. Mix the wet ingredients into the dry ingredients and knead, either in the stand mixer on the lowest speed or with your hands in a large bowl, until the mixture forms a dough.

Continue to knead for another 7 minutes in the mixer or 10 minutes by hand on a floured work surface until smooth and elastic.

Place the dough in a clean bowl, cover with a damp tea towel, then leave to rise in a warm place for a couple of hours until doubled in size, or you can leave to rise overnight in the fridge.

Make the filling. In a medium-sized bowl, cream the butter, cinnamon and sugar together with a wooden spoon. Set aside.

Knock the dough back by plunging your fist into the middle, then tip it out onto a lightly floured surface and briefly knead.

Roll out the dough to 20 x 30cm. Evenly spread the filling over the surface of the dough, then spread the marmalade over the top.

Holding the long end, roll the dough into a tight sausage and cut it into approximately 12 rounds, each about 2.5cm thick. Space the buns out evenly in two large cake tins, allowing them room to spread. Cover with a damp tea towel and leave the buns to rise again for around 30 minutes.

Meanwhile, pre-heat the oven to 200°C/Fan 180°C/Gas Mark 6.

Bake the buns in the cake tins in the oven for around 20 minutes. Leave in the tin, spread over the marmalade glaze, and serve warm.

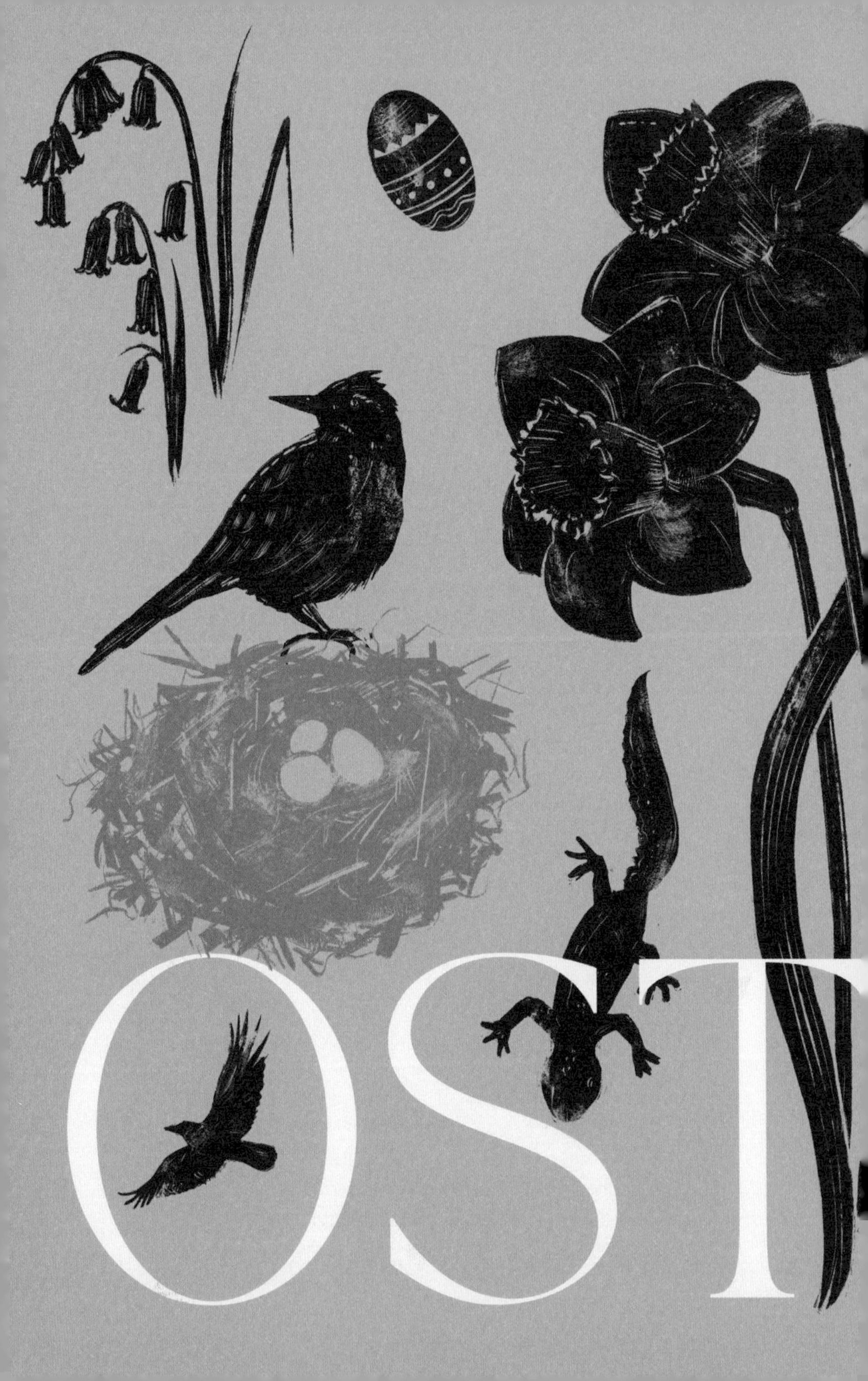
OST

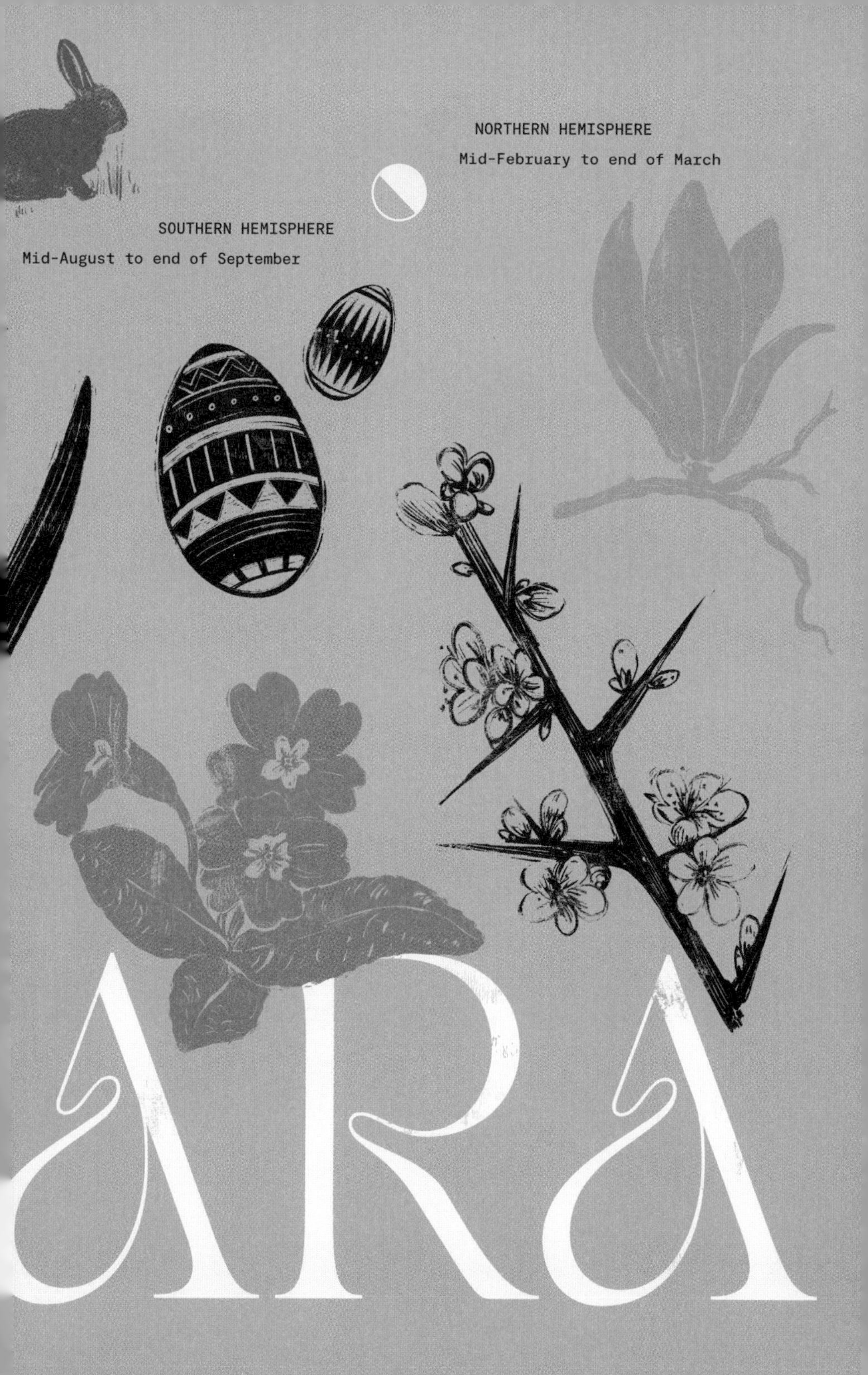
NORTHERN HEMISPHERE
Mid-February to end of March
SOUTHERN HEMISPHERE
Mid-August to end of September
ARA

SPRING STIRRING

In the Celtic Wheel of the Year, the festival of Ostara marks the Vernal Equinox, when night and day are of equal length once more. Just as it begins to feel like Winter will never, ever end, nature gives us some small but certain signals that Spring is stirring beneath the earth.

Ostara signifies balance as we begin the shift back towards longer, lighter days. The mercury is gradually rising, and the flowers and leaves are beginning to bud. This is a time of transition between Winter and Spring and offers a myriad of magical contradictions: birdsong and storms, daffodils and mud, a new dress under a Winter coat.

Lengthening days gather apace and slowly but surely the weather improves, corresponding with rising energy levels – in nature, and in ourselves as part of nature. A rebirth is underway as we begin to awaken from Winter once more. There's something so cathartic about preparing yourself – and your home – for Spring after a long, cold Winter.

Ostara is traditionally associated with fertility, renewal and rebirth. The Christian celebration of Easter has many links with Ostara and several contemporary traditions have evolved from Celtic symbols. For instance, the hare, linked to the moon, rebirth and immortality, is a traditional Celtic symbol for Spring, and is thought to be where the Easter bunny comes from. Another well-known Easter symbol is the egg – representing fertility, growth and balance, apt for the Spring Equinox – which has links with the Celts as well as Christianity.

These days, I like to do something small but special to mark the Vernal Equinox, whether making a pavlova full of Spring flavours or visiting the botanical gardens here in Edinburgh to spot the ever-growing signs of Spring. Many such signs can be found all around you during this six-week period if you just look for them, starting with daffodils and primroses.

> SUDDENLY THE WORLD SEEMS GREEN AND GLORIOUS. SUDDENLY EVERYTHING SEEMS POSSIBLE. SPRING IS STIRRING.

Seasonal Celebrations at Home

Ostara coincides with the Spring Equinox, a time of equilibrium, with day and night being of equal length before the light takes over and the sun's ascendence towards Beltane and Summer begins. All that building energy, light and life signals the opportunity for fresh starts, plans and projects. This is a time to be outdoors as much as possible, to shed a layer or two, to bring nature inside, to celebrate the first of the new season produce: a taster of all the seasonal goodness to come.

Bring Spring Indoors

I love to bring nature inside in any season, but something about taking home those first Spring flowers is extra special. You can 'force' blossom by bringing it inside: a kindly neighbour might have magnolia you can prune, or your local florist might have branches of seasonal blossom. Make sure your branches' buds aren't too tight, and prune them on a warmer day so the indoor heat does not shock them. Look up the best pruning method for the tree or shrub in question, but generally try to take branches from denser areas and around the back; and always cut at an angle rather than straight-on.

Cut a deep cross in the bottom of each of the branches to help with water uptake, then pop them into a big old preserving jar filled with a little water and leave them to blossom somewhere light and warm but away from direct heat and sunlight. Change the water each day and re-cut the stems to keep your branches healthy and lengthen their vase life.

Or you can go miniature with tiny flowers of grape hyacinth, narcissi or fritillaria. Distributing single stems of these smaller flowers in a variety of wee receptacles makes a small posy go a long way and provides more visual impact on a table or mantelpiece. I'm forever collecting Victorian ink bottles and cheap stoneware pots at car boot sales and flea markets for this purpose. As with branches, change the water frequently to keep your thirsty Spring flowers fresh.

Spring Sorting

Spring cleaning might sound like a cliché, but my urge to declutter is almost instinctive. I find cleaning quite therapeutic; a good clear-out at the start of the season can be incredibly cathartic and makes your environment and mindset ready for the season ahead. I usually wait for school holidays, when I have the time and headspace to deep clean and declutter, but if you're short on time, committing to one small task each day (or week) is helpful to chip away at bigger tasks, maintain momentum and feel a daily dose of fulfilment. Even if it is just one drawer, corner or surface, it's a start. I often focus on clothes, as I start to consider my lighter layers, decide what to donate and check if anything needs mending. When Gran came to visit when I was growing up, one of her jobs was the mending pile – as a dressmaker there was nothing she didn't love to fix or patch. There are lots of mending tutorials available online – such as Japanese sashiko – that add prettiness as well as functionality to past-their-best pieces. There can be fewer simple-yet-rewarding pleasures than tackling a spot of mending with a cup of tea and good audiobook for company.

Spring Watch

Incorporating a little nature into every day is good for the soul. At this time of year I like to engage in some morning mindfulness with birdsong. It's unavoidable where I live, on the third floor next to a huge silver birch tree. Listening to their cheerful music growing daily is an impossible-to-miss sign of Spring for me and never fails to make me feel more positive. When you wake, keep your eyes shut and carefully listen to the sounds around you. Follow the call and response of the birds as you gradually unfurl your body, feeling each of your limbs and stretching your fingers and toes.

I also find changing my route to work a helpful strategy in the mornings. It might add another five minutes to my journey, but altering my surroundings just slightly makes me more attuned to the environment. Even swapping the side of the road I walk on makes me notice new things – from the first daffodils by the roadside to the blackthorn-covered hedges. Try it; you might be surprised by what you see with a simple change of perspective.

Decorating for Ostara

I used to often decorate eggs with Mum, Gran and my brother. Gran collected onion skins and naturally dyed her eggs long before it was an Instagram trend! I have lovely memories of afternoons sat at the kitchen table making our eggs into characters with wool plaits and painted smiley faces. After the effort that went into making them so pretty, I never wanted to take part in 'pace eggin', the Scottish tradition where you decorate your egg then roll it down a hill!

To make natural dye, you can use all sorts of store-cupboard ingredients. There are lots of natural dye colour charts online to guide you to create a whole rainbow of colours. My favourite ingredients to use are spinach, which makes a pastel green, and chopped beetroots, which make a pink dye. Experiment with different spices such as paprika and turmeric, or other vegetables such as red cabbage.

To naturally dye your eggs, place uncooked eggs (white shells are best) in a pan and cover with at least 5cm of water. Add 2 tablespoons of vinegar per litre of water and your chosen natural dye ingredients. Simmer the eggs and dye ingredients until they reach your desired shade, checking on the colour of the eggs every so often – mine take around 30 minutes to achieve a pastel hue. Take off the heat and remove the eggs with a slotted spoon. Air dry on a wire rack. I like to make two different colours (pink and green – my favourite) and display the eggs in mismatched bowls on the table.

RHUBARB, WHITE CHOCOLATE & GINGER PAVLOVA

The first shoots of forced, early Spring rhubarb are usually available in greengrocers and shops in the lead-up to Ostara. Its bright pink stems are a cheerful antidote to grey days and provide vital colour and flavour during the 'hungry gap' between the end of Winter fruit and vegetables and Spring's glut. This rhubarb, white chocolate and ginger pavlova combines a sweet chocolate cream and fiery ginger-poached rhubarb filling in a marshmallowy pavlova and can be decorated with Easter eggs for Spring celebrations. I tend to make the pavlova the night before, leaving it to dry out overnight in the oven, and then make the filling and assemble it the next day for a celebratory lunch.

SERVES 8

For the pavlova
3 large free-range egg whites
175g caster sugar
½ tsp cornflour
½ tsp white wine vinegar

For the compote
200g rhubarb
60g caster sugar
1 tbsp crystallised or stem ginger, finely chopped
Juice of ½ lemon

For the chocolate cream
50g white chocolate
150g double cream
Chocolate eggs, to decorate (optional)

First, make the pavlova. Pre-heat the oven to 160°C/Fan 140°C/Gas Mark 3 and line a baking tray with non-stick baking paper (if you want, you can draw a roughly 20cm circle on it as a guide by drawing around a cake tin).

Put the egg whites into a large bowl and whisk with an electric hand-mixer or in a stand mixer on the fastest speed until stiff; they should be able to hold their shape when you turn the bowl (carefully!) upside down.

With the mixer on a medium speed, gradually add the 175g caster sugar in generous teaspoonfuls, continuing to whisk until the sugar has dissolved (the mixture should no longer feel grainy) and the mixture forms stiff peaks and looks smooth and shiny.

In a bowl, mix the cornflour and white wine vinegar together until smooth, then fold into the meringue mixture, being careful not to knock out all the air.

Place half the meringue mixture onto the middle of the lined baking tray, spreading it into a roughly 20cm circle. Fit a piping bag with a rose nozzle and fill it with the rest of the meringue mixture. Pipe equally spaced 'nests' of smaller circles around the outside of the pavlova.

Slide the meringue onto the middle shelf of the oven and reduce the heat to 140°C/Fan 120°C/Gas Mark 1. Bake for 1–1¼ hours, or until the pavlova is sturdy – it should easily peel away from the paper – and it is a creamy, pale pink colour (rather than white).

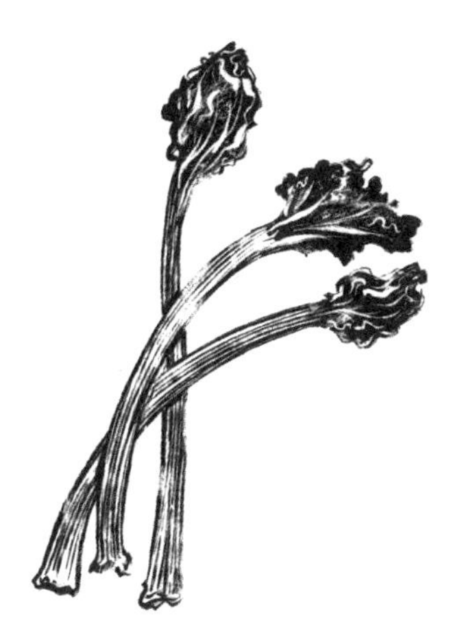

Once it has cooked, turn off the oven and leave the pavlova to cool in the oven for a few hours, or overnight.

When you are ready to make the compote, remove the pavlova and pre-heat the oven to 220°C/Fan 200°C/Gas Mark 7. Cut the rhubarb into 2.5cm pieces (they look big, but this is so they hold their shape when baked) and place in an ovenproof dish. Cover with the sugar, ginger and lemon juice, stir and tightly cover with foil. Bake for 30 minutes until the rhubarb starts to give but still holds its shape, then leave to cool.

Meanwhile, melt the white chocolate in a heatproof bowl set over a small pan of simmering water, making sure the bowl doesn't touch the surface of the water. Stir the chocolate regularly until half of it is melted, then remove from the heat and set aside for a few minutes to let the residual heat do the rest. Stir until smooth and set aside to cool.

In a new bowl, whip the cream until it just starts to become stiff. Fold the cooled chocolate through it (if the chocolate is not sufficiently cooled it will make your cream grainy).

Fill the pavlova centre and nests with the cream and add some of the rhubarb on top (reserve the juice to dilute in a delicious cordial!), then decorate with the chocolate eggs, if you like. Serve immediately with the rest of the rhubarb alongside for guests to help themselves to more.

SETTING A SPRING TABLE

My annual ritual of setting the table to welcome the Vernal Equinox makes me mindful of the small, seasonal changes and new beginnings all around us as we emerge from Winter's grip. The festival of Ostara is the high point of many Spring celebrations, taking place on the Spring Equinox when the sun appears directly above the Earth's equator, between 19 and 21 March every year. Ostara, adopted from Anglo-Saxon traditions, has historical associations with other religious festivals: for instance, Jewish Passover is usually the first full moon after the Vernal Equinox, while Christianity defines Easter as the first Sunday after the full moon on or after the Equinox.

For each of the festivals in the Celtic Wheel I enjoy setting the table for a simple, seasonal celebration. I have fond memories of helping decorate and set the table at home when I was growing up. Seasonal decorations, napkins and even crockery were hidden away until their moment to shine, a tradition that I continued after leaving home. Bringing them out only for brief spells around these seasonal transition points makes them more special to me.

The ritual of creating a tablescape is just as important to me as what's on the plate. In my opinion, making the effort and including even just a little decoration – a simple linen napkin, a single candle, a posy of flowers – is an easy way to elevate the everyday. Even if it's 'just' for yourself, setting the table is a centring ritual. It reminds us that eating nurtures the soul as well as the body.

I do take particular care to decorate around each of the celebrations in the Celtic Wheel of the Year and often leave the decorations up for a week or two afterwards, a gentle reminder of the change of the seasons.

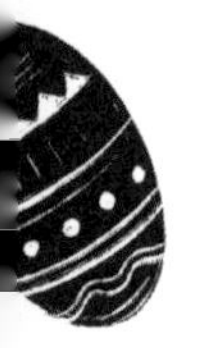

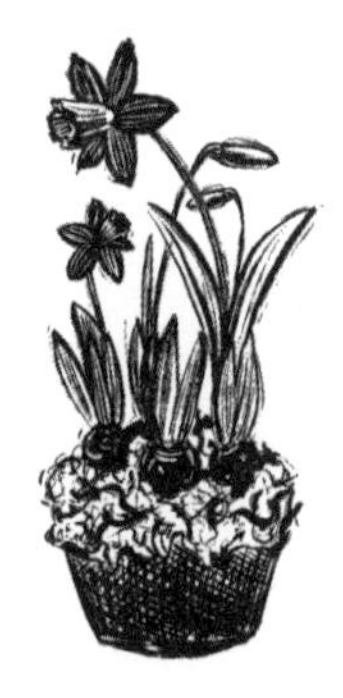

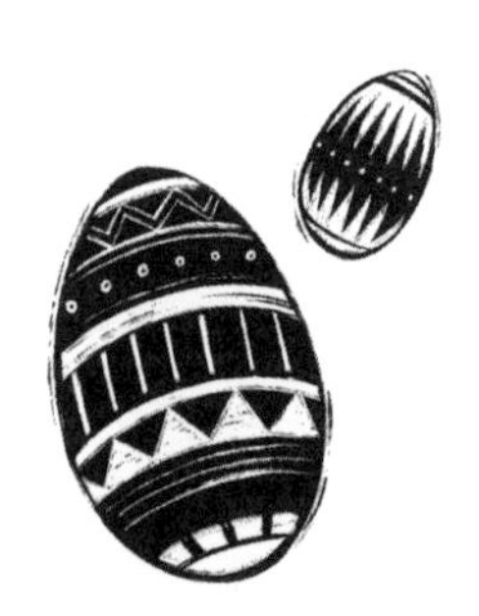

CREATING A SPRING TABLESCAPE

First, I decide on my colour palette. I am often inspired by the colours of nature itself – this time is synonymous with sugared almond shades so I usually go for dusky, springlike pinks and soft yellows. I start most of my tablescapes with flowers, which I source from sustainable, locally grown flower farms. In past years, blush-coloured narcissi, frilly ranunculi and branches of blossom have all featured. I usually go for one central arrangement: a simple jam jar, maybe tied with a ribbon, is sufficient to store your arrangement and allow it to sing.

I like to use a solid-coloured tablecloth as my base layer and have built up quite a collection of linens over the years. You can create your own table runner and napkins (see page 48) to further customise your décor and add pattern and texture.

When dressing the table I like to use mismatched pieces from my vintage collection to add personality. Layering plates is a good way to create visual interest, then I add tonal napkins, simply folding them and tying them with sparkly twine or ribbon. I decorate with a stem of foraged greenery or a pine cone on top, and instead of place setting cards, use traditional brown card luggage labels decorated with pastel calligraphy names.

Then it's time to add height: taper or dinner candles are your friends. I use vintage candle stick holders – again, mainly mismatched – that I have collected over many years, alongside miniature jam jars or crystal glasses. You can source coloured candles from so many places, especially independent sellers online. My favourites are naturally dyed beeswax candles. Everything feels instantly cosier as soon as I've lit them.

My chairs are all sourced from charity shops, and my mid-century kitchen table is well-loved. Lastly, I finish things off by adding faux fur blankets and throws over the backs of chairs to add cosy texture and warmth.

You could add a woodland bulb display (see page 55) and serve wild garlic pesto pasta (see page 53) to complete your Ostara celebration.

A Note on Sourcing Props and Thrifting Tips

- Always be on the lookout as you never know what you will find. I once wheeled a mid-century drinks trolley all the way from one side of Edinburgh to the other.
- Popular pieces can have a hefty price tag – be ready to haggle, unless you're in a charity shop.
- Know your location: be prepared to pay a wee bit more for quality and authenticity at specialist antiques fairs.
- Always snap something up when you see it if you love it. I'm still haunted by the mid-century deckchairs I once had my eye on, which I left while I looked round the shop.

Make Your Own Table Linens

Making your own linens is easier than you think – and often cheaper too. You can completely personalise your fabrics to fit your colour scheme and create a bespoke table setting. Cotton is easiest to work with as well as care for, and will age beautifully. Patterned fabric has a 'right' side (where the pattern is printed, usually a smoother surface) and a 'wrong' side (usually a rougher texture and slightly faded appearance), but if you are using something like linen this will be the same either side.

I'm often on the lookout for Liberty London's ditsy print Tana Lawn fabrics in the remnant bin of my local fabric shop, which has come up trumps on several occasions. It is usually a fixed, pre-cut length, but it's amazing what you can do with a scrap or two!

TABLE RUNNER

A table runner is a simple way to update your table if you don't want to use a full tablecloth or want to layer different textures and patterns over a tablecloth, and gives you a protective surface for hot dishes and candles. Again, please use whatever size fabric you already have to avoid scraps, or use my guide for measurements below. This craft is best made using a sewing machine rather than by hand, unless you are very patient.

YOU WILL NEED

Measuring tape
Fabric, washed and pressed – see method for dimensions
Iron and ironing board
Pins
Thread that matches the fabric
Sewing machine

Measure the width and length of your table. Divide the width by three, then add 2cm to allow 1cm hem allowance on either side. For the length, decide how much overhang you want at either end of the table, then again add 2cm to allow 1cm hem allowance at each end.

Now, start the double fold hem. Fold over one edge of the fabric 5mm to the wrong side. Press with the iron along the hemline. You will probably have to do this in stages for the long edge of the fabric.

Fold over the new edge 5mm to the wrong side again to create a double fold. Press again. Pin into place. (If you're not a confident sewer, you can also tack the fabric into place: roughly sew with large, temporary stitches in a contrasting thread you can remove later.)

Now it's time to sew: set up your machine as per the manufacturer's instructions. Starting with the long side, straight stitch forwards, then backwards for a couple of stitches on the wrong side of the fabric, then stitch all the way down the length of the runner as close as you can to the fold line.

Repeat for the other three sides to complete your runner.

Press your runner again and position it in the middle of the table.

NAPKINS

Making your own napkins is a fun way to start bringing a more personal touch to your table setting, and you can make four from just a metre of fabric. Here I've used a double fold hem to keep your napkins looking neat and so that they wash and wear well. You could also machine stitch your napkins, but I will explain how to slip-stitch by hand as I know not everyone has a sewing machine at home and this is a useful, discreet stitch to learn. A slip-stitch is created by sewing along the fold of the hem, just lightly picking up the threads on the other side. Alternatively, you could do a running stitch in a thicker contrast thread (such as embroidery or sashiko thread) to make a feature of the stitching and make this craft really simple.

To make napkins in your desired size, you could choose a favourite napkin you already have and measure it; mine was 45 × 45cm and I added a 1cm hem allowance but do use the fabric that you have – it's not the end of the world if your napkins are rectangular, or slightly smaller than 45cm as this avoids ending up with scraps (though if you do, there's a fun project on page 69).

YOU WILL NEED

- Fabric, washed and pressed – see method for dimensions
- Measuring tape (optional)
- Scissors
- Iron and ironing board
- Pins
- Thread that matches the fabric
- Needle

Cut your fabric into four even squares: fold it into quarters, pressing after each fold, then cut along the creases. (I used 94 × 94cm for four 45cm napkins with a 1cm hem allowance either side.)

With your fabric right side down, take an edge and make a fold to create a hem: fold the fabric 5mm in on itself to the wrong side. Press with the iron along the hemline.

Fold the new edge 5mm over towards the wrong side to create a double fold and press again. Pin into place.

Thread the needle with a double thread: pass a long piece of thread all the way through until the ends meet and tie a knot at the end to make a big loop.

Sew the hem with a slip-stitch: with the wrong side of the napkin facing you, insert the needle into the hem fold to make a stitch. When you bring the needle out of the fold, pick up a thread or two of the fabric on the right side of the napkin and pull the thread through. Exactly where the last stitch ended, place your needle back inside the fold of the hem.

Repeat all along the edge until you reach the end. Finish off by putting your needle through the last stitch at the back a few times, then trim the thread.

Repeat to sew the hems for the other three edges; the corners will overlap and be slightly bulkier, but that's OK.

Press the napkin. Repeat the process for the other three napkins.

Alternatively, you could use a sewing machine and straight stitch all the way round the double hem to secure it in place, remembering to finish off your stitches at the start and end.

Simple Variations

- Don't be precious about matching your napkins. Use up scraps of fabric in complementary colours to make a mismatched set.
- You could add a trim to the napkin – go wild in the haberdashery with pompoms, beads or fringing.
- Have fun folding and arranging your napkins. For Ostara I like to fold napkins into bunny ears around a decorative egg: fold a napkin in half to make triangles, then fold over several times to make a long thin strip. Wrap around an egg and tie with a ribbon at the top to make two 'ears'.
- Embroider initials or a motif onto your napkin: draw your design using an erasable pen and use a small hoop and embroidery thread. You could use an embroidery kit; or experiment with the embroidery setting of your sewing machine to make a repeat pattern such as hearts or flowers.

Seasonal Celebrations of Nature

Around the Vernal Equinox there is always something new to observe, to bring joy and to ground you in the here and now. In Scotland, the novelty of it being light past 6 p.m. is enough of a thrill, never mind spotting the first jolly faces of daffodils or enjoying the abundant blossoms beginning to bud on the trees. The first UK lockdown began in the lead-up to Ostara; in Scotland we were allowed out to exercise once a day. I found our daily walk was transformative: from the joy of watching the first narcissi open at the start of the lockdown to the wisteria arriving as restrictions eased, I'd never needed to notice nature more.

Many animals begin to come out of hibernation, the warming earth a signal to them, and us, to become more active once again. Rabbits can be spotted above ground, searching for food in fields (and even in the city – I once saw some rabbits in Edinburgh's central park, the Meadows, in spite of its busyness). The trees are still bare, so it is easier to spot woodland wildlife too – from voles to deer.

The first butterflies of the year can be seen on milder days. If you have a garden, it is well worth leaving a patch of plants to do its own thing. The likes of nettles and brambles provide shelter and food for emerging, sleepy insects.

The distinctive white flowers of the blackthorn, small clusters close to the branch and lethal thorns, fill the hedgerows – take serious note of its positioning as its flowers will become sloe berries, which are harder to spot in the Autumn. Yellow primroses spring up in woodlands and on banks just before abundant wild daffodils, surely the most iconic flower of Spring. Soon, a carpet of wild garlic (ramsons) forms, which you will smell long before you see it. They are best foraged as young shoots, before their white flowers appear in April when they become stronger and more flavoursome. Look out for the first growth of new needles on pine trees, so you can forage pine tips for preserving and making pine sugar (see page 167). Bluebell leaves push through the soil in February and begin to unfurl in milder areas as early as March – look out for them in ancient woodlands.

Millions of migrant birds now arrive in the UK – try to spot them with a pair of binoculars and use a guidebook to identify their features. (I found my battered but beautiful copy of the *Observer's Book of Birds* in a charity shop.) Shelter and dark coloured clothing usually help by giving you more time to identify them. Try photographing or sketching them to capture the memory.

Breeding season has begun for some species of birds: rooks in the woods and gannets at the coast. The call of skylarks can be heard on coastal marshes as they compete for mates, those with the broadest song repertoires usually seeing greatest success. Many artists, including the Lakes poet Wordsworth, have been inspired by their song.

In woodlands you can also hear the distinctive wooden sounding call of the cuckoo, though they are very difficult to spot; while grey herons will be building their nests in colonies – listen out for their noisy beaks which create a surprisingly loud clattering.

Many freshwater invertebrates begin to emerge in streams and ponds around Ostara. This is amphibian breeding season, so warmer days are likely to draw these amphibians from their hiding places. On lakes and other bodies of water grebes can be spotted courting – a surprisingly balletic display that I've observed even on Blackford Pond, in the middle of the city here.

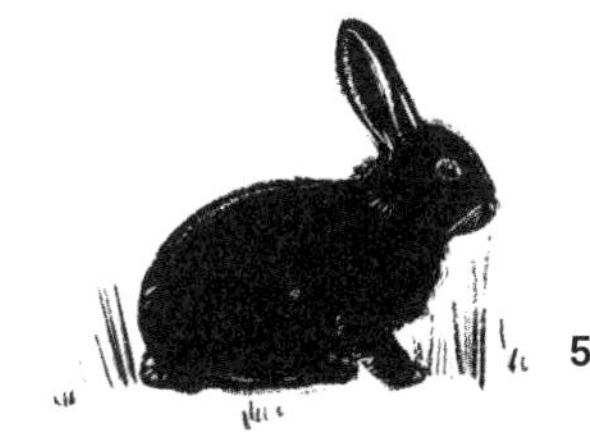

OSTARA WOODLAND MAKES

As the season turns with the Spring Equinox, the first flurry of woodland floor activity begins, particularly spectacular in ancient woodlands as nature bursts into life once again: surely a tonic after the Winter months. As the trees are generally still bare, the light filters through to the undergrowth with ease. Over this six-week period between Ostara and Beltane, nature transforms.

In Scottish folklore, creamy yellow primrose flowers are associated with fairies. The so-called 'fairy cup' is seen as lucky, bringing blessings and protection to the household. As one of the first Spring flowers, it is a herald of good luck and constancy. The wild garlic beginning to carpet the forest floor is also associated with luck – it was thought to bring strength to those who consumed it, and the bulb was even used later in medicine. Its Latin name, Allium ursinum (bear garlic), refers to the fact that brown bears used to love eating wild garlic; it is known colloquially as bear's leek.

Evergreen gorse flowers between January and June but is usually at its most fragrant, with its distinctive scent of coconut, around Ostara. Gorse was often burnt as fuel as it has a high percentage of natural oils; its flammable nature and bright flowers meant the plant became associated with the sun, fire, light and its life-giving powers. It's easy to see why the fast-growing and hardy shrub represents resilience and optimism.

Bluebells are native to western Europe. They have been found in ancient woodlands for thousands of years and have long been linked with fairies in folklore. Many different stories set in woodlands involve dark fairy magic. One story goes that if you pick a bluebell, you will be led astray by fairies and wander lost for all time. Another even says that if you hear a bluebell ringing you will be visited by an evil fairy and will die soon afterwards.

Here are some ideas to capture and preserve the spirit of the woodland, so that you can be transported back to its calm with a wee slice of everyday nature. Remember to forage responsibly and to ask the landowner's permission before you go picking. Take sparingly from each patch and – if there is a significant amount – certainly no more than a third of what you find in each area, leaving plenty for the wildlife.

WILD GARLIC PESTO

As it is so abundant and easily identified (its aroma giving away its position), wild garlic is a great introduction to foraging, perfect in pesto and salads. If you can't find wild garlic in the great outdoors, ask your greengrocer or the provider of a local veg box. Wild garlic is milder in taste than standard garlic and makes a pleasingly green pesto that practically sings of Spring. Use as you would a standard pesto: to generously coat pasta, dress salads or flavour soups.

MAKES APPROX. 300G

200g wild garlic
Boiling water, for blanching
Generous glug of olive oil
75g toasted nuts (pine nuts are classic but can be expensive – I use walnuts or pecans)
50g Parmesan or other hard cheese (choose one that's vegetarian, if making this for veggies), grated
Juice of ½ lemon, or more to taste
Sea salt and black pepper

Rinse the wild garlic carefully to remove any mud and beasties and place it in a very large heatproof bowl. Boil the kettle.

Completely cover it with boiling water for 1 minute to blanch it; this takes away the raw taste and makes it wilt.

Drain the wild garlic in a colander, giving it a good shake to remove as much of the moisture as you can.

Transfer the wild garlic to a food processor and blitz to a bright green paste.

Add a good glug of olive oil, the toasted nuts, grated cheese and lemon juice and blitz again.

Taste and add a little salt and pepper and more lemon juice, if needed. Taste again and decant into a bowl, then use as desired.

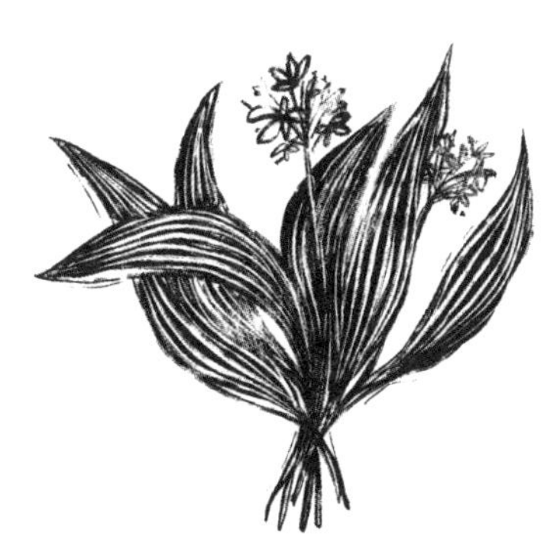

GORSE PETAL TEA

Gorse flowers are edible: they have a tropical, herby taste that echoes their fresh, grassy, coconutty scent that is deliciously springlike. Use as you would any edible flowers, for example to decorate cakes, stir through salads or infuse in syrups. You can also make gorse petal tea with the flowers.

YOU WILL NEED

Long, thick gloves, for foraging
Cotton bag
Tea towel
Boiling water
Teapot and cup

Forage for gorse flowers on a sunny Spring day. Wearing long, thick gloves – and watching your arms! – pick the gorse flowers from above waist height: you want to take just the yellow flowers, so carefully pinch them – you don't want the green bit at the top or the spiky leaves. You need to gather at least a few handfuls of petals in your cotton bag – which takes longer than you think but beautifully engages all the senses.

Gorse flowers provide shelter to lots of insects, so when you get home, lay the flowers out on a tea towel, preferably outside, so they can make their escape!

To make fresh gorse petal tea, boil the kettle. Take a handful of the flowers (roughly 1 tablespoon) per person and squash them in your hand to bruise them.

Place the petals in a teapot, cover with boiling water and leave for about 10 minutes to infuse.

Strain into cups and enjoy.

Tip

If you don't want to make the tea immediately, you can dry out the gorse petals. Just leave them spread out in a single layer on a tea towel in a warm, dry spot for 1–2 days (not the kitchen as it is usually too damp). The flavours will intensify so you will need less in your tea – around half the amount as fresh, but experiment and see how you prefer the taste. The dried flowers will last for many months in an airtight container, though their flavour will fade over time.

WOODLAND BULB DISPLAY

I like to bring bulbs indoors, particularly my favourite miniature Tête-à-Tête daffodils, which always remind me of Granda who loved and tended his each Spring. I like to make a display of bulbs on my mantelpiece as a simple celebration of Spring: a reminder of woodland calm, and of this comforting memory of my grandparents' garden. Once your bulbs have bloomed, let the foliage die back, then they can be planted outside for next year.

YOU WILL NEED

- Newspaper or old sheet
- Spring bulbs in pots with green shoots (from a florist or garden centre) or small Spring bulbs grown for indoor use, such as grape hyacinths, fritillarias or narcissi
- Dry, stubby paintbrush
- Sustainably sourced moss (available from florists)
- Glasses, jars or pots, to display the flowers
- A plant mister spray or small jug, for watering
- Fairy lights
- Dried bracken, pine cones and other foliage
- Florist's wire

Cover a work surface with the newspaper or sheet.

Remove your Spring bulbs from their pot. (This is easier with dry soil, so do not water just before starting.)

Gently remove the soil from around the roots and start teasing them apart until you can separate each bulb from the roots of the rest – this requires patience and a gentle hand.

Remove the soil from around the roots, brushing them with a dry paint brush if needed. You can wash them if you like.

Place some dry moss in the bottom of your chosen receptable.

Arrange your bulbs by gently placing them into the moss.

Once you are happy with the arrangement of the bulbs (don't over-crowd them), cover the roots with moss. The bulbs might look a little floppy at first but once the roots settle in, they will begin to perk up and grow upwards towards the light.

Fill your plant mister with water and spray the moss so it is damp, or use a jug and pour in just enough water to make the roots and moss damp – but not where the roots join the bulb as this can rot.

Arrange your bulb jars in the area you want to decorate. Grouping them in odd numbers is aesthetically pleasing.

Wind your fairy lights around them; they are particularly pretty shining through the jars from behind.

Finish the display by arranging pieces of bracken, pine cones and other foraging finds around the jars. You may need to wire them in place, onto the shelf or to the fairy lights themselves. Play around with them until you have an arrangement you like – you're trying to create the impression of a wild woodland floor, so don't be too precious.

Regularly mist or lightly water the moss to keep the flowers healthy.

Support the flowers with twigs if they are getting leggy and top heavy, tying them in place with a little twine.

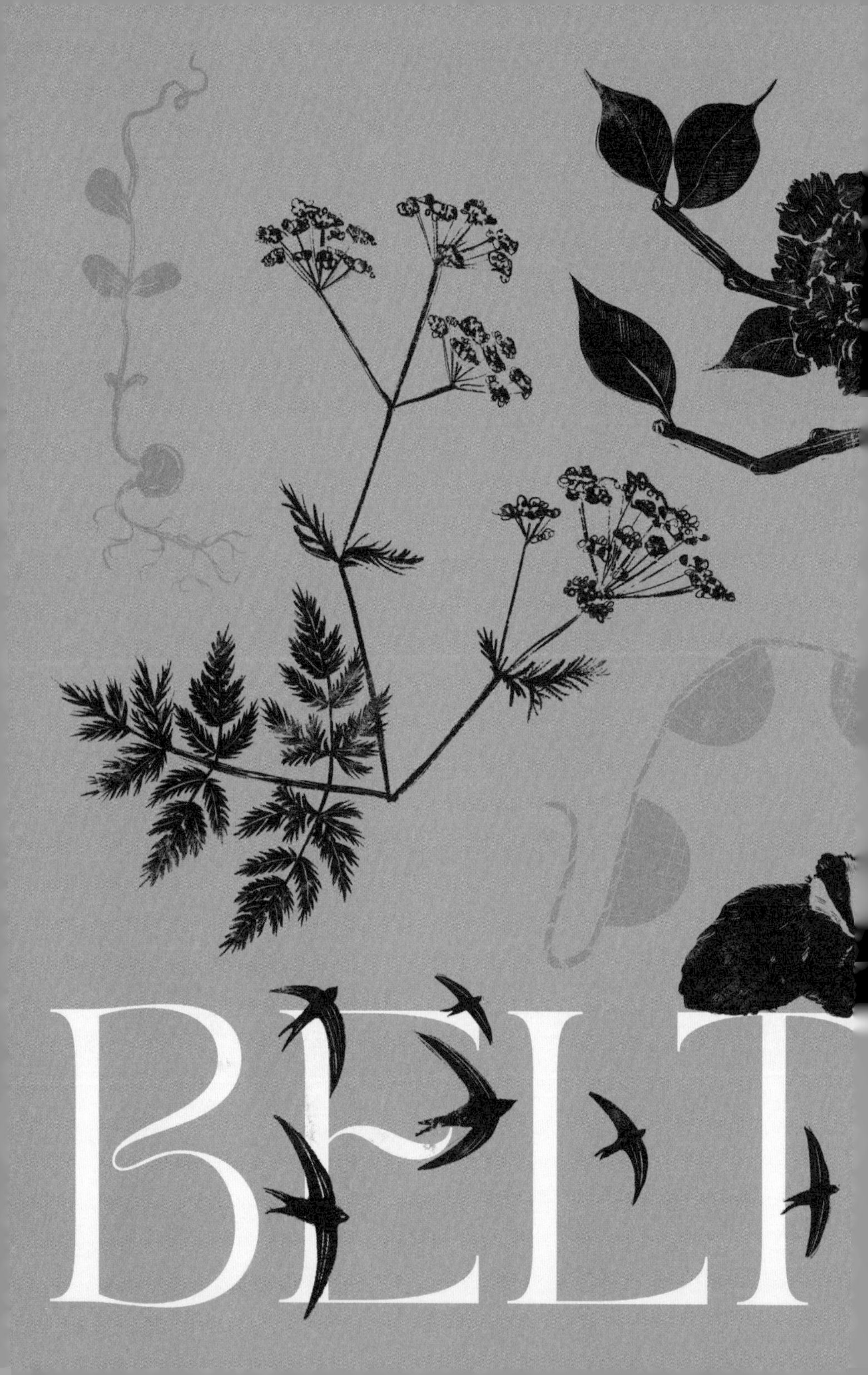

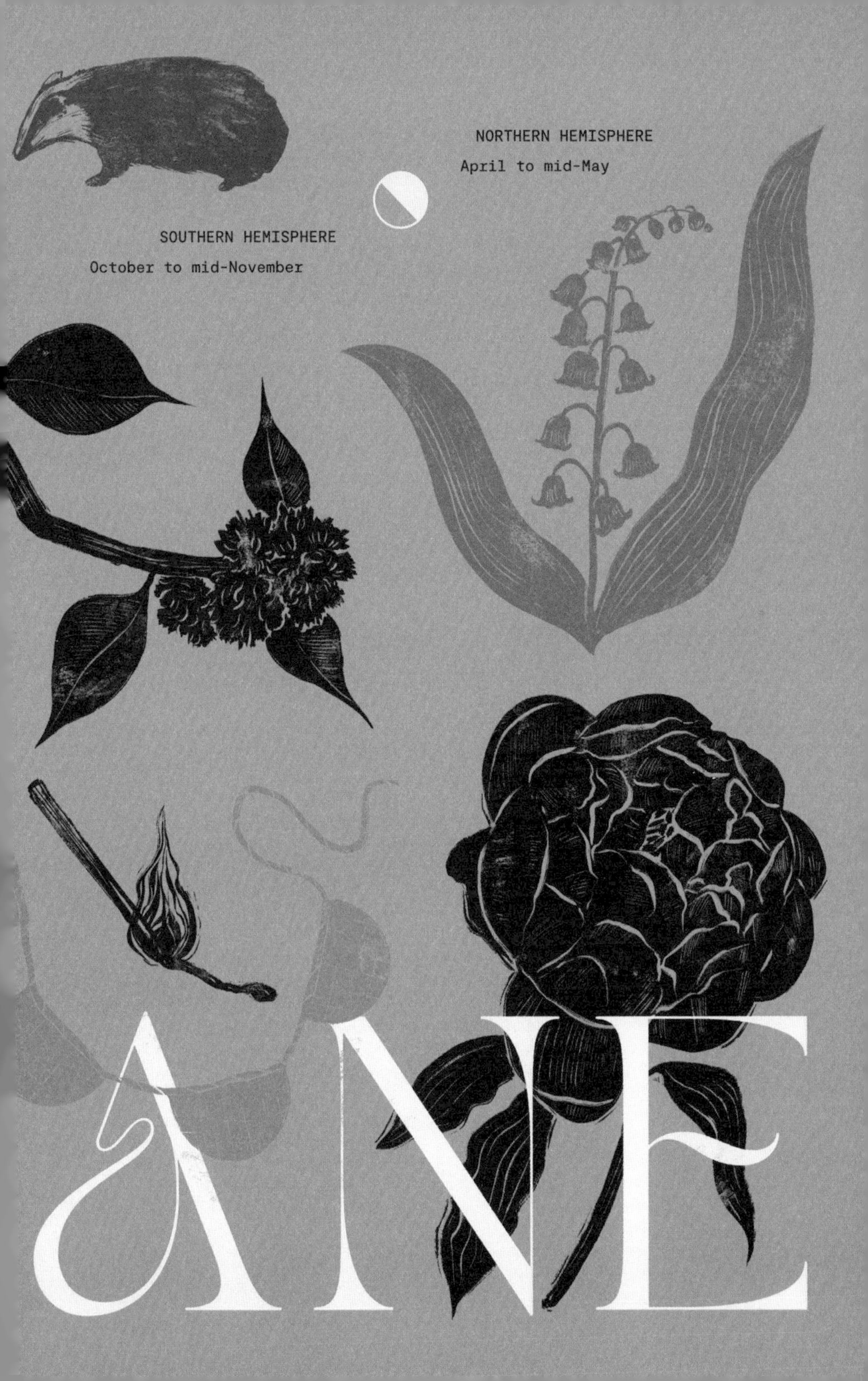
NORTHERN HEMISPHERE
April to mid-May
SOUTHERN HEMISPHERE
October to mid-November
ANE

CELEBRATING LIFE

Beltane celebrates the halfway point between Ostara, the Vernal Equinox, and Litha, the Summer Solstice. It takes place on 1 May and is traditionally a time of fire and feasting to welcome the return of the light as the days get longer. The name 'Beltane' comes from Gaelic for 'fires of Bel' (a Celtic god) and heralds the beginning of the farming year, a time of hope, growing abundance and community. These days, the biggest Beltane celebrations in the UK are held in Edinburgh with bonfires at the top of Calton Hill that are lit in the evening and brightly burn until dawn, symbolising light, fertility and creativity.

In the Celtic Wheel, Beltane marks the beginning of Summer. Earlier than its meteorological counterpart, this time has always felt to me like a countdown to Summer: May was the month of exams in Scotland (now a month of marking as a teacher!) while Dad's birthday is at the end of the month; Beltane always seemed to signal the start of holiday celebrations as we approach the Scottish school break in June. As a student at the University of St Andrews, we celebrated with the 'May Dip': running into the North Sea at dawn – typically after staying out all night – which was considered to 'cleanse' you of academic sins.

Ancient festivals and holidays with dancing, singing, cake and flowers have long taken place at the start of May across European cultures. In England, the May Queen is crowned on May Day, with dancing around the maypole and ribbons. An old May Day tradition that has seen a delightful resurgence in recent years is the annual ritual of leaving a small posy of flowers on the doorstep of friends' and neighbours' homes to celebrate the new season.

> AT THIS TIME NATURE IS CELEBRATING LIGHT AS WELL: TRADITIONALLY, IT WAS THE END OF THE 'HUNGRY GAP' IN THE HARVEST CALENDAR WHEN THE NATURAL WORLD SEEMED ABUNDANT AT LONG LAST.

This six-week period is particularly flower-packed. Blossom is bursting into life, with the cherry blossom bringing cheer to the daily commute: a reminder to take our time.

Visit the countryside and you will find the hedgerow is awash with white hawthorn – aptly named May blossom – and cow parsley lining fields and roadsides. In the garden, the ephemeral blooms of lilac and lily of the valley are all the more precious for their fleeting beauty. Their scent alone evokes seasonal joy as high Spring meets early Summer.

Seasonal Celebrations at Home

Beltane was traditionally the start of the farming year, as light and warmth gather apace. The corresponding explosion in nature offers so much to cherish as the sun gets higher in the sky, new produce arrives and the flowers abundantly bloom.

Cherry Blossom Syrup
Beltane coincides with the peak of blossom season. The world's most iconic cherry blossom celebrations take place in Japan, where locals engage in hanami or 'flower viewing' – a traditional ritual of enjoying the ephemeral blooms of the cherry blossom with picnics and outdoor parties during its short, three-week season. In Scotland, 'gean', wild or bird cherry trees, were thought of as unlucky, even referred to as a 'hagberry' in Scots. Perhaps this is because they were rare – solo trees appearing on the edge of woods – so seeing one would be quite a sight. These days, I like to pack a simple, seasonal picnic and head to our local park, the Meadows, where cherry trees line the walkways.

I was inspired to make my own cherry blossom syrup after tasting cherry blossoms with blackcurrant ice cream at nearby Elliott's Studio, run by cookbook author Jessica Elliott Dennison. The blossom imparts a floral, fruity, almost almond-like flavour. To make a small bottle of syrup, dissolve 100g caster sugar in 200ml water and boil until reduced and syrupy, then infuse a large handful (around 20g) of cherry blossom petals for a few hours. Taste it, then infuse for longer if you want a stronger flavour. Strain into a sterilised bottle and store in the fridge. Drink as a cordial, diluted with sparkling water, or use to drizzle cakes, bakes and ice creams. You can try this with other Spring flowers such as gorse or lilac too!

Planning Summer Adventures

If living seasonally has taught me anything, it's that I can live in the moment as well as look forward to the next season, particularly at liminal times of year like Beltane. It's around now that I like to plan a Summer adventure or staycation to build excitement for the longer, lighter months that now feel close enough to taste. Having a date in the diary, a note in the calendar to count down towards, gives me that school Summer holiday feeling of anticipation. Since the pandemic, many of us are holidaying closer to home and redefining the phrase 'change of scene'; we don't have to go far to give ourselves a needed reset. My favourite place for a spot of R and R is Guardswell Farm, just over an hour away from Edinburgh. We stay there in a simple larch cabin, nestled in the woods and looking out over the Carse of Gowrie. It's where I let myself completely slow down and simply watch the changing sky, spot lambs and hares in the fields, and prepare a seasonal supper in the minimal kitchen with ingredients fresh from the farm. S'mores and sunsets finish the day, and I almost always fall asleep reading. Just thinking about it makes me feel calm: I hope you can find a place like this and make it your own, as well as recreate some of its magic at home. Anticipating our visits, I sometimes do a mindful ritual of boiling a kettle on the wood burner, Guardswell style, and making a slow cup of tea: preparing the leaves, stirring them in the gradually boiling water, steeping and straining, hugging my hands around my favourite mug and listening to my breathing slow.

Sow Some Seeds

It's time to start planting, even if you only have an indoor garden like me. I've still got my name down for an allotment in Edinburgh (six years on the waiting list, and apparently at least another six to go) so I won't be sowing seeds directly into the earth any time soon. However, you can grow a surprising amount in a wee space like a windowsill. As long as it gets plenty of light, you're good to go. Growing pea shoots is easy all year round, but something about their sweet, green freshness is perfect for late Spring and early Summer. Technically, pea shoots are just the young tips of the pea plant; these days you can even buy them in supermarkets but growing your own is much more fun – not to mention tastier – and they are ready to eat in just a few weeks.

You will need a shallow container, around 10cm deep, that has drainage (seedling trays are ideal but you could make holes in any receptacle – even a used punnet or tray from your food shop). Soak some pea seeds in water overnight. Fill the container with about 7cm peat-free potting compost, then water liberally and allow to drain. Sow the seeds generously, about a centimetre apart. Cover with a 2cm layer of potting compost and water again. Place your container on a sunny windowsill. Turn it every few days (the pea shoots will grow towards the light) and check if the soil is still moist, watering as soon as it begins to feel dry, and more frequently once the pea shoots start to appear. You can start harvesting your pea shoots as soon as they are around 10cm long – after two to three weeks – and they can give you multiple harvests; simply trim with kitchen scissors just above the first leaves. Don't let them get too tall as they will lose their sweet flavour and pleasant texture. As the pea shoots are young, they are filled with nutrients and lovely to top risottos, pasta dishes and anywhere you would use salad leaves.

Seasonal Produce

The kitchen can breathe a sigh of relief after the 'hungry gap' and the arrival of Spring produce such as asparagus and Jersey Royal potatoes – their highly seasonal nature makes them even more delicious for their short-lived appearance. Beltane is the beginning of the exciting culinary shift towards Summer abundance, a taste of the lighter flavours of the season to come. I find the best way to let these ingredients sing is to serve them simply:

asparagus lightly fried and finished with lemon zest and toasted almonds. New potatoes boiled and simply served with a knob of butter and sprinkling of sea salt. Herbs are plentiful in May; for a simple supper, roughly chop mint and basil and toss with lemon juice and olive oil to dress a burrata salad with the first, freshly podded peas of the year and your home-grown pea shoots. In May, the first Summer fruits start to arrive in time for the first al fresco meals of the season. These precious early berries might need a little help getting the most of their flavour; macerating new season strawberries with a little elderflower cordial can give them a lift and floral sweetness.

Flower Spotting (and Eating)

It's around Beltane that gardens and green spaces start coming into their own, and doors to country estates are open again after their Winter hibernation. A dream day out for me in Spring and Summer involves a country walk or a trip to a local garden, strolling and flower spotting. Each week seems to bring new flowers to see and fresh Spring colour. Bonus points if there's a tearoom nearby, or bring a flask of tea to enjoy outdoors. My favourite garden to visit is Malleny Garden in Edinburgh's southern suburbs; there are bluebells and wild garlic in the woods, alliums and the first peonies emerging in the garden, and highlighter-pink pelargoniums in the glasshouse.

ROSE & STRAWBERRY VICTORIA SPONGE

To get a taste of Spring gardens at home, you could make your own floral Victoria sponge. Baking with rose can divide a crowd but used sparingly it gives a delightful sunny twist to baking staples – such as this rose and strawberry Victoria sponge. Here the sponge is infused with rose extract, then sandwiched with homemade jam and light-as-air rose buttercream (or if you prefer whipped cream, then a few drops of rose extract will add a floral note).

SERVES 8

175g unsalted butter
175g caster sugar
1 tsp rose extract
3 large free-range eggs
175g self-raising flour
1 tbsp water
100g strawberry jam
Dried roses or rose petals, to decorate (optional)

For the buttercream

50g butter
110g icing sugar, plus extra to decorate
1 tbsp warm water
¼ tsp rose extract

Pre-heat the oven to 180°C/Fan 160°C/Gas Mark 4. Grease and line two 18cm round tins.

With a wooden or silicone spoon, cream the butter and sugar with the rose extract in a bowl until light and fluffy.

Add the eggs, one at a time, along with a little of the flour and the 1 tablespoon of water.

Fold the remaining flour gently into the mixture.

Evenly divide the batter between the two tins, then bake in the oven for 25–30 minutes, until the sponges are golden and a skewer inserted in the middle comes out clean.

Set the sponges aside to cool a little, then remove them from the tins and cool completely on a wire rack.

Make the buttercream by creaming the butter and icing sugar with the warm water and rose extract in a bowl until fluffy and white in colour – about 5 minutes.

Assemble the Victoria sponge: place the first sponge on your serving plate, then cover the top with a layer of jam (warm it in the microwave to loosen if you need to) spread almost to the edges.

Add the buttercream on top, again spreading almost to the edges. Place the second sponge on the top and dust with icing sugar, decorating with the dried rose petals, if using. Allow the icing to set for around 30 minutes, then slice and serve with a pot of tea.

BELTANE PICNIC

The festival of Beltane is a symbolic casting away of darkness, letting in the light once again. This time has been fêted in different forms in Ireland, Scotland and the Isle of Man since the Iron Age, people coming together to celebrate Summer's return, the start of the farming year and nature's rebirth.

As with many of the festivals in the Celtic Wheel, Beltane celebrates light and fire. Symbolically, fire is a purifying element: the ritual lighting of the Beltane bonfire representing the growing power of the sun and regeneration following Winter's darkness. Traditionally, families would walk around the fire, some people even jumping over it for good luck. Animals would similarly be purified, being led around – and even over! – the fire before heading to the fields newly protected.

Another Beltane tradition was the extinguishing of the hearth fire and candles and lighting of the new, communal bonfire, usually on a nearby hill, where food was also cooked and enjoyed together, and subsequently used to rekindle each of the individual hearths. This was regarded as a moment of sacred community connection and bonding. Greenery would also be displayed as decoration, and Beltane 'bannocks' (flat, savoury cakes made with oatmeal and cooked on a griddle) were traditionally served to guests.

Beltane has been long associated with courting, match-making, fertility, creative community and abundance. At one time, Beltane celebrations took place on the peak of Edinburgh's group of hills, an extinct volcano that looks like a sleeping lion called Arthur's Seat, with bonfires and beacons. The tradition died out for many years, but the practice has recently revived in Scotland, mainly thanks to the School of Scottish Studies at the University of Edinburgh. The world-renowned Beltane Fire Festival in Edinburgh takes the spirit of the festival and now attracts thousands of visitors to another of Edinburgh's vantage points, Calton Hill, every year for ritual displays and performances. A torchlit procession starts at the National Monument and goes clockwise around the hill, led by the traditional May Queen to the sound of drums. There is a performance of the death and rebirth of the Green Man or Oak King, who represents the Summer part of the seasonal cycle in various folk traditions, and he and the May Queen light a huge bonfire. Visitors gather for music, dancing, food and drink.

HOSTING YOUR OWN BELTANE CELEBRATION

Today, I like to hold my own Beltane celebrations, lighting a fire in the stove at home, heading to the beach for a bonfire or to picnic outdoors. At some point I will climb Arthur's Seat to be outside: it never fails to put things into perspective. The tiny figures below and the memory of the centuries of Beltane celebrations in this very place remind me of a long-ago narrative and sense of belonging.

My favourite way to celebrate is a picnic in the garden (usually my parents'). A simple garden picnic, at your house or a friend's, is a lovely excuse to make a delicious spread of picnic treats and maybe even decorate. Picnics combine good food, good company and the great outdoors. If the weather has other ideas you can always picnic on the living room floor as I did with a group of friends one soggy Summer in St Andrews – it was even more memorable for it.

I have many fond memories of family picnics from my childhood: exciting days out in the big city, eating soggy tomato sandwiches in the car, or braced behind wind breaks in the dunes of West Sands in St Andrews; or closer to home – snacks eaten hurriedly in the garden between games. Picnics don't have to be just for special occasions; my friends and family know I am rarely without some sort of picnic, snack, back-up snack or on-the-go eats ready to share. It's the feeder in me – Gran and Mum are entirely to blame for instilling this instinct to share and nurture through food!

The word 'picnic' originates from the French *pique-nique*, a meal where guests provided a share of the food each. This shared ritual of preparing the picnic can be just as enjoyable as the event itself: organising with others what you are going to make, gathering ingredients and preparing your contribution, filling flasks, digging out the picnic blankets and loading a basket or two with treats.

SETTING THE SCENE

If you can, set up your picnic spot beneath some trees so you can hang decorations such as bunting or garlands, and shelter from the Spring breeze if you need.

Bunting adds a sense of occasion to an otherwise standard picnic. Rag bunting is an easy make that is as simple as it sounds, doesn't involve sewing, and is a fun way to use up fabric scraps. For the more confident sewer, there's also scalloped bunting (see page 70).

You will need a few blankets, cushions and something to put your spread on: I use a couple of vintage butler's trays I thrifted in charity shops, but you could use anything raised such as old garden crates. You could even ask your guests to bring their own cushion and blanket to make themselves at home and create an even comfier setting.

A fire pit or fire log is an easy way to recreate a Beltane bonfire in the garden without the commitment to making your own pyre, and probably (definitely) safer. Follow the instructions carefully and make sure to keep children and pets well away from naked flames and hot surfaces. Summer is on the way but the Scottish saying goes 'ne'er cast a clout 'till may is oot' (don't put your warm clothes away until May is over), so a wee fire is ideal to chase away an evening chill.

Place jars of flowers on the makeshift tables and hang jars of flowers or banners from the trees using string or twine. Hang them at different heights for maximum impact. Just remember to take your string down afterwards so no wildlife gets hurt.

You could ask your guests to bring an item to eat each – just make sure you share a list of who is bringing what so that you don't end up with all bread and no dips, or vice versa. For seasonal picnic ideas, see pages 71–5.

RAG BUNTING

Rag bunting or ribbon garlands (probably sounds more glamorous) is a great, no-sew way to use odds and ends of fabric – I can't be the only one who finds them difficult to throw away! I have a whole box of fabric scraps that I have kept from my childhood, which is perfect as my palette was pretty consistently pink, purple and green. Some would say little has changed. You don't have to use scraps though; you could buy ribbons for this purpose – the great thing is that you don't have to be precious, and the more rustic and random the better.

YOU WILL NEED

- Fabric offcuts or ribbons, as many as you can get your hands on (if making the bunting using ribbons, start from step three)
- Cord, string or twine
- Scissors
- Measuring tape

Tear your fabric offcuts into roughly 2cm strips (cut a notch and simply tear to create a rough edge).

Cut the strips to a roughly similar length – around 15cm is a good length.

Cut the cord, string or twine to your desired length of bunting (measure the space where you are going to hang it, then add a little more for tying).

Tie the middle of each fabric strip onto the cord, string or twine, equally spacing them along its length. You can make the bunting as full as you like: more strips will make for fuller bunting. If you are using different colours and fabrics try to alternate them for the best effect.

SCALLOPED BUNTING

When it comes to decorating, I favour curved shapes, scallops and circles, so this scalloped bunting is a contemporary twist on staple bunting. It's a similar process to the traditional triangles, but you are sewing curves instead of points (slightly trickier but even prettier).

YOU WILL NEED

Plate or bowl (as a template for the scallop shape)
Cardboard
Pencil or pen
Scissors
Fabric pen or tailor's chalk
Cotton fabric, washed and pressed – see note for dimensions
Scissors
Pins
Sewing machine
Thread to match your fabric
Measuring tape
Knitting needle
Iron and ironing board
Bias binding, in a coordinating colour, washed and pressed – see note for dimensions

First, draw around the plate or bowl onto the cardboard, then cut out to make a semi-circle template. Keep in mind that this includes a 5mm seam allowance, so the final scallop will be slightly smaller.

Using tailor's chalk, draw around the template close to the raw edge of the wrong side of your fabric. Repeat all along both raw edges until you have drawn your desired number of scallops (e.g. for nine scallops, you will need eighteen semi-circles). Cut out all the scallops.

Place two scallops right sides together and pin along their curved edges. Leave the straight edges open. Repeat for the other scallops.

Thread your sewing machine and set to a straight stitch.

Sew a scallop together 5mm in from the raw edge, following the gentle curve of the semi-circle as you go, going slowly and stopping every few stitches to pivot the fabric (remember to backstitch at the start and end). Repeat for the remaining scallops.

Carefully make small cuts from the raw edge towards the line of stitching all around the semi-circle of each scallop. This will help your fabric curve when you turn it inside out.

Turn each scallop inside out, so that the right sides are now outside. Use a knitting needle if any bits are being stubborn and won't lay flat, and press with a hot iron.

Place your bias binding on a flat surface and arrange your scallops in between along its length, evenly spacing them out with some empty binding at each end to hang your bunting. Press and pin into place.

Using a straight stitch, sew along the length of the binding to sew it together and encase each of the scallops inside the binding, remembering to backstitch your sewing at the start and end.

Trim the ends of the binding on the diagonal to make a neat finish.

Give your bunting another press, then hang it up!

Note

For 2m bunting with nine 14cm-diameter, 7.5cm-deep scallops spaced roughly 1cm apart and with 30cm either end for hanging, you will need roughly 144 × 17cm fabric and 2m bias binding.

BEETROOT PANCAKES

These are my nod to the bannocks of my ancestors and the tattie (potato) scones that my gran used to make, fried with leftover mashed potato and served with a cooked breakfast – but these are a lighter alternative that still nods to the root veg flavour. You can get beetroot powder online and from health food shops, but you can leave it out if you can't find it.

MAKES APPROX. 12

100g self-raising flour
20g oat flour (blitz 20g rolled oats in a blender)
1 tsp caster sugar
¼ tsp sea salt
2 tsp beetroot powder
6 tbsp milk, plus extra to loosen, if needed
1 large free-range egg
Butter, for frying

Mix the flour, oat flour, sugar, salt and beetroot powder in a large bowl.

Whisk the milk with the egg in a jug, then pour into the flour mixture, a little at a time, whisking to combine until you have a thick, 'dropping' consistency; add a little milk if the mixture seems too thick.

Put a frying pan over a medium heat, and melt a knob of butter.

Working in batches, add tablespoons of the mixture to the pan and cook for 2–3 minutes, or until small bubbles form on the surface.

Using a spatula, gently turn the pancakes and cook them for another 2–3 minutes until set and starting to turn golden.

Tip

- Make a cream cheese topping to go with your pancakes: whisk 100g cream cheese with a tablespoon of fresh thyme and season to taste. Loosen with a little milk if the cream cheese is particularly thick.
- Transport the topping in a Tupperware box and serve at the picnic with another sprinkling of herbs or a slice of pickled onion or beetroot to add a sharp contrast.

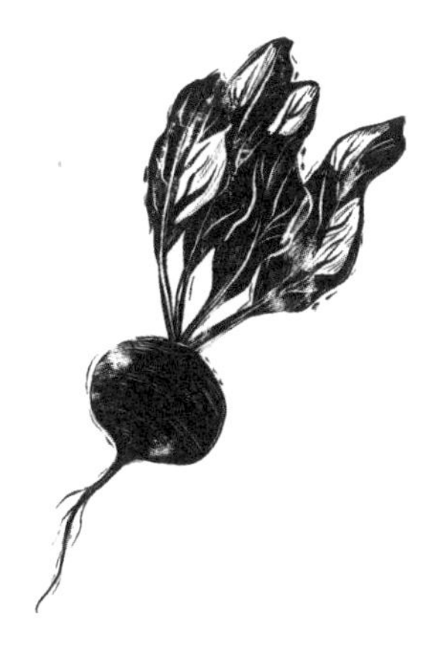

PESTO PALMIERS

Palmiers are wee French pastries that look impressive but are easy to make with shop-bought puff pastry, and can be made either savoury or sweet by adapting the filling. Their name comes from their distinctive shape – translating as 'palm trees'. They're also known as 'elephant ears'.

MAKES APPROX. 48

Plain flour, for dusting
375g packet ready rolled puff pastry
8 tbsp pesto (or the wild garlic pesto on page 53)
6 tbsp any grated cheese (I like Pecorino – choose a vegetarian version if serving veggie friends)
Milk, for brushing

Line two baking trays with greaseproof paper.

Dust a work surface with flour and unroll the puff pastry. Roll out with a rolling pin in one direction to make it just a couple of millimetres thick.

Spread the pesto across the surface of the pastry.

Scatter 4 tablespoons of the grated cheese over the pesto.

Roll one of the long sides of the pastry into the middle, then roll the other side into the middle so the two spirals meet. Press them together so the pastry sticks.

Turn over the rolled pastry so the join is underneath and place on one of the baking sheets. Chill in the fridge for 30 minutes.

Pre-heat the oven to 220°C/Fan 200°C/Gas Mark 7.

Remove from the fridge, then cut the pastry widthways into 5mm slices using a sharp knife to make individual palmier rolls.

Lay the palmiers flat on the greaseproof paper on the trays and lightly flatten them by rolling over them with a rolling pin.

Brush the palmiers with a little milk, then sprinkle with the remaining 2 tablespoons of grated cheese and bake for 10–12 minutes until golden and crisp.

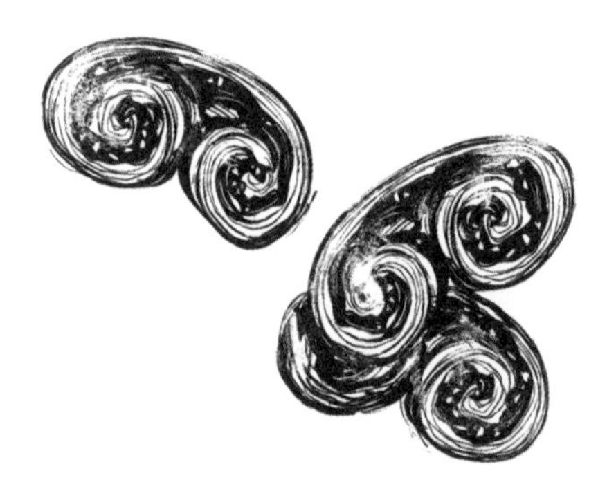

SCONES

When I was growing up, scones often featured in family picnics and days out, even in my school lunchbox – there was barely a week that went by without a fresh batch being made at home. Their nostalgic comfort takes me straight back to cosy car picnics and teatimes at Gran's house, served still warm from the oven and oozing with butter. Here is my basic family recipe.

MAKES 12

- 225g self-raising flour, plus extra for dusting
- ¼ tsp salt
- 25g caster sugar
- 50g butter, diced
- 70g dried fruit and/or nuts of your choosing
- 100ml milk, plus extra for brushing

Pre-heat the oven to 220°C/Fan 200°C/Gas Mark 7 and line a baking tray with greaseproof paper.

In a large bowl, mix the flour, salt and sugar. Add the butter and use the tips of your fingers to very lightly rub it in until the texture resembles breadcrumbs. At this stage, mix in your fruit and/or nuts.

Add the milk to the flour mixture a little at a time, bringing the dough together with your hands. You might not need it all – you want the dough to be firm, not wet.

Gently knead the dough on a lightly floured work surface, then press it into a disc about 2cm thick.

Using a 5cm scone cutter (or a glass if you don't have one) cut your scones into rounds. Make sure you press straight down and pull straight back up, otherwise your scones will rise in a twisted fashion.

Gently knead together the offcuts and continue cutting out scones.

Place your scones on the baking tray, brush the tops lightly with milk and bake for 12 minutes, until golden brown.

ALMOND & CHERRY COOKIES

Another feature of family picnics were 'jam buns': a biscuity sponge cake with fresh jam in the middle, which became chewy and caramelised when cooked. This recipe is my take on them, a cross between a chewy macaroon and an amaretti biscuit with a pool of cherry jam in the middle. I've used cherry jam as cherries aren't in season in the UK until July, but they'd be lovely later in the year with half a fresh cherry baked into the middle.

MAKES 12

- 60g ground almonds
- 85g caster sugar
- 1 free-range egg white
- ¼ tsp almond extract
- 1–2 tbsp cherry jam

Pre-heat the oven to 180°C/Fan 160°C/Gas Mark 4 and line a baking tray with greaseproof paper.

In a large bowl, mix the ground almonds and caster sugar.

In a separate bowl, whisk the egg white and almond extract with a fork until starting to froth. Add to the almond sugar mixture and stir with a wooden spoon until you have a soft dough.

Take a small spoonful of the mixture at a time and roll into a ball – wet your hands to help if it is too sticky.

Place your cookies on the baking tray, spacing them well apart (they will spread) and use a thumb to make an indent in the middle of each.

Fill the holes with a pea-sized amount of jam (if you overfill them, the jam will bubble out and burn). Bake for 25 minutes, until golden and cooked through.

Leave to cool on the tray, then pack up for your picnic.

JAM JAR ETON MESS

Portable puddings are the order of the day, and nothing says Summer like Eton Mess: bashed up meringues, fresh fruit and whipped cream. I've gone for a recipe inspired by Scottish cranachan, the traditional pudding with oats, cream, crowdie soft cheese, raspberries and honey. I use frozen raspberries as it's still a little early for their fresh counterpart – but you can also make this later in Summer with the first, fresh seasonal fruit.

SERVES 4

150g raspberries
150ml double cream
1 tbsp clear honey, plus extra to taste
50g meringues (shop bought, or adapt the pavlova recipe on page 42), broken into pieces
A handful of oats, toasted in a dry frying pan until golden

First, make a compote with the raspberries: put them into a medium-sized pan.

Heat over medium–high, stirring regularly, until the raspberries soften and cook through. Remove from the heat and transfer to a bowl to cool, then chill.

Whip the cream to soft peaks in a bowl and sweeten with a tablespoon of honey.

Fold the broken meringue pieces through the cream mixture.

Sample the raspberry compote and add honey, 1 teaspoon at a time, to your taste (it should still be sharp enough to cut through the rich cream and sweet meringue).

Ripple most of the compote through the cream mixture. Decant into jam jars.

Top with another drizzle of compote and the toasted oats. Firmly screw on the lids and pop in your picnic basket.

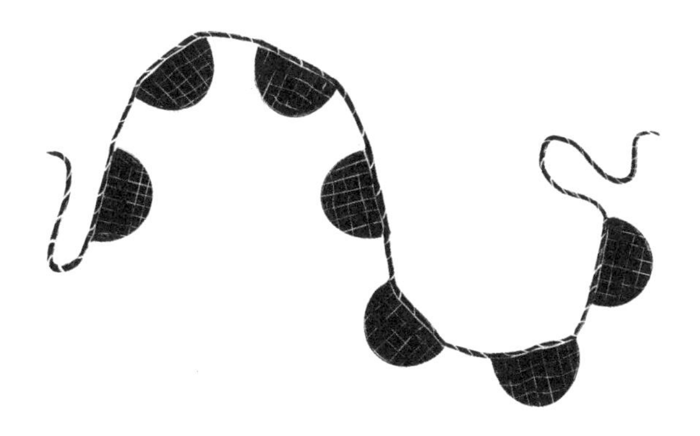

At Beltane, nature is fuelled by the growing energy resulting from the Earth tilting closer towards the sun. In Britain it's a white-out in the hedgerows with blossom in full bloom. Wild garlic and wood sorrel still carpet the forest floor in green with the last of the bluebells and distinctive purple or white violets poking through. Violet flowers traditionally symbolise love and can be found in damp, shady patches such as beneath hedgerows or at the foot of trees in the forest. Heavy dew and the golden hour make a magical combination, so head out early with your camera to catch the unmatched dawn light.

Beltane brings warm evenings, an ideal time to see wildlife up close, from a covered position. Common lizards, who live in grassland and sand dunes, are now in their mating season. Badger cubs peep out from their setts at twilight. And you might even spot baby hares frolicking in open fields. Hedgehogs emerge from hibernation to breed; they produce several young babies called hoglets between early Summer and Autumn. Beetles also emerge; look out for the wasp beetle and cardinal beetle with their vibrant, warning colours of yellow and red respectively.

This is a time associated with new life: birds are in full nesting mode, protecting eggs, then feeding newly hatched chicks. Listen out for their demanding calls and watch from a safe distance. Birds of prey can be seen hunting above motorways: the kestrel hunts in daylight, making it one of the easiest to see with the naked eye.

Beltane also sees the return of swallows, swifts and house martins: watch them swoop across blue skies on warm days. Their high-pitched song heralds Summer's arrival. The three birds are very similar and easily confused – especially when moving quickly. Swifts are dark brown with a short, forked tail, while swallows have blueish feathers, a long, forked tail, a red throat and a white tummy.

House martins are the smallest of the three, with shorter wings and a pure white tummy. The haunting song of the nightingale can also be heard in the south of the UK; they tend to hide in the undergrowth, so you are likely to hear but not see them.

Nesting seabird colonies, particularly gannets, kittiwakes (listen for their distinctive, onomatopoeic call) and puffins, are a fascinating sight as they, too, become more active. Peregrines are the UK's fastest bird and are often seen on the coast throughout the UK and in rivers as the days lengthen.

Similarly, the onset of warmer weather induces many fish to breed, such as minnows, carp and sea trout. Male sticklebacks flaunt bright red undersides and green backs to attract a mate and can be spotted in ponds, rivers and lakes, waving water over eggs with their tails to provide a regular supply of oxygen and, when threatened, fiercely fight potential predators.

Orcas can even be spotted in small numbers near the clifftops of Orkney and Shetland, visiting from Iceland and Norway to hunt seals.

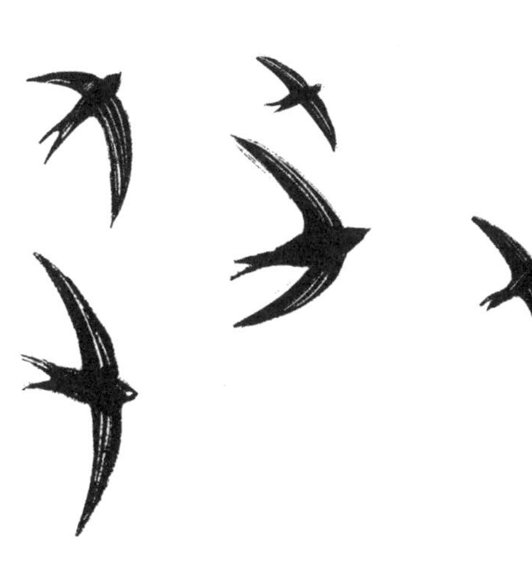

BELTANE SEASONAL FLOWERS

Decorating with seasonal flowers has long been a part of Beltane and May Day celebrations, including the anonymous gifting of a Spring posy. In recent years, this lovely gesture has seen a resurgence thanks to social media and the hard-working florists promoting British blooms across the country that are ripe for the picking.

The small size of a posy arrangement means that you can make the most of the season's delicate blooms, arranging complementary colours and textures. Nature gives us lots of white flowers along with pastel shades of pink and purple. You could even consider the colour of door you will be placing your posy on, for maximum coordination… Or maybe that's just me!

I always keep an eye out for small vintage vases, glasses and bottles for Beltane posy making. Many everyday objects are great for repurposing, too; small glass bottles or jam jars work perfectly – just wash them in warm water to remove their labels and make sure they're scrupulously clean, as flowers require crystal-clear water. Finishing your posy with a ribbon in a coordinating colour can cover all manner of imperfections if your receptacle is less than perfect.

SEASONAL FLOWERS

Lily of the valley
(*Convallaria majalis*)

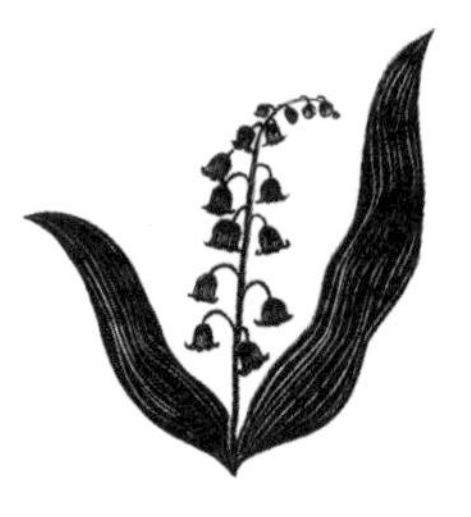

The tiny, white, bell-shaped flowers are synonymous with Beltane – their fragrance transports me straight to late Spring. This is tricky to grow and can be obtained from local florists. Its season is extremely short, but its miniature charm more than makes up for this lack of longevity, and it is surprisingly hardy for something that looks so delicate. When bought, it often arrives with the roots attached; trim as close to the root as you can, on the diagonal, then use the longer stems in the centre of the posy.

Lilac
(*Syringa vulgaris*)

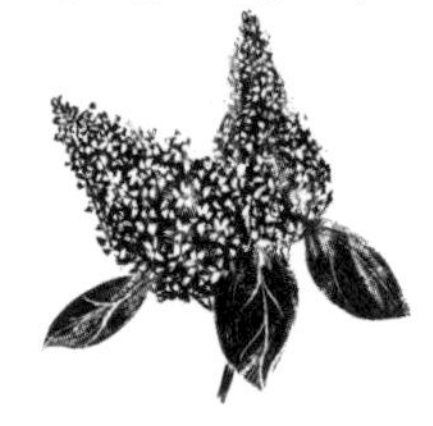

Believe it or not, lilac is actually part of the olive family. Its scent is sweet and heady, making it a fragrant option for cutting. The flowers are even edible and can be infused in syrups, honey or sugar. As well as the signature, expected lilac colour, white and deep purple varieties can be found. As lilac is a shrub or small tree, it has only a slim, woody stem and doesn't last long in a vase, so remove most of the large leaves to direct water to the flowers. Searing the stems also helps: place the ends in boiling water for thirty seconds, then put them in a bucket of cold water for a few hours.

Peony
(*Paeonia*)

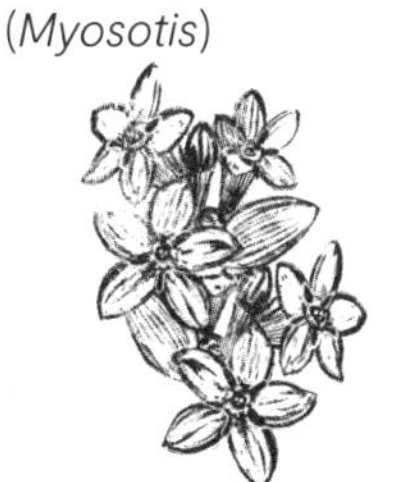

The peony has been ubiquitous on Instagram for the last few years, but it's easy to see why; its large, blousy, ruffled blooms are incredibly photogenic. My parents used to have a deep red version in their garden, and I associate Beltane with its brief season and watching its transformation from impossibly tight bud to frilly flower to pool of fallen petals. In a small arrangement, just one peony is needed to add a little luxury.

Forget-me-not
(*Myosotis*)

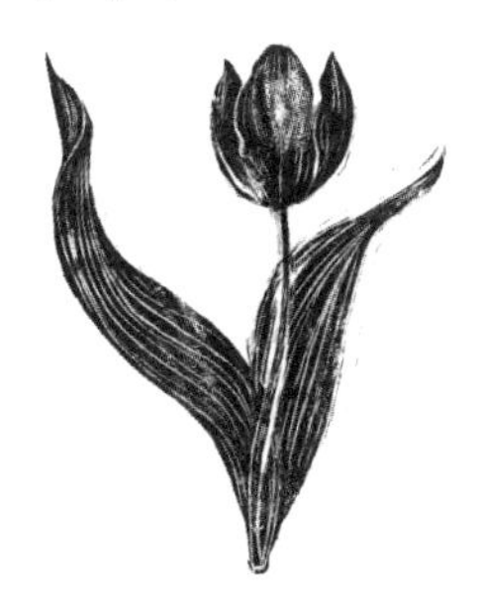

The tiny blue flowers of forget-me-not bloom from May and can last all the way through Summer. You can also find pink and white varieties. The flowers are so delicate and vivid and look stunning en masse. Forget-me-not has long stems so is good for arrangements and even produces sweet little seedpods along the stems once it has gone over. Forget-me-not is said to represent purity and fidelity, hence the name.

Tulip
(*Tulipa*)

There are so many different varieties of tulip these days, the parrot or fringed tulips even competing with peonies for drama and impact, as well as a whole palette from deep, almost black purple to purest white with an array of vivid colours in between. Supermarkets are getting much better at stocking British tulips at a reasonable price. It is the only cut flower that grows in the vase, and I love how tulip arrangements evolve over a few days as a result. If your tulips are too droopy, add a copper coin to the bottom of the vase to perk them up.

Ranunculus
(*Ranunculus*)

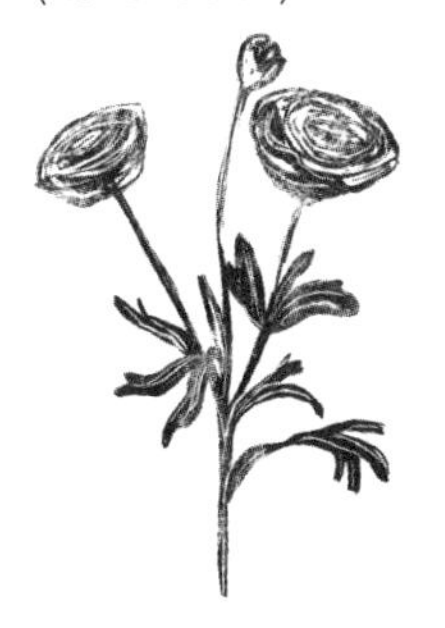

Ranunculus blooms from Spring to early Summer, with distinctive, numerous clusters of petals and a gorgeous range of colours from soft pastels to vivid brights. You can even get very ruffly, peony-like varieties. I love the warm tones of reds, peaches and pinks together. It lasts well in a vase if cut as the buds are beginning to open and you can just see the soft petals (this is called 'marshmallow stage', which I love). Wild buttercup is part of the ranunculus family and in Latin ranunculus means 'little frog'.

ARRANGING A POSY

For something of this scale, my guiding principle is to have one feature or focal flower, two or three smaller stems to complement it and some greenery or blossom.

YOU WILL NEED

Flowers
Scissors
Small bottle, glass or vase
Greenery or blossom
Florist's wire
Ribbon

Lay out each stem in a row on a flat surface so you can see the different colours, heights and textures and envision the design.

Condition the flowers by freshly cutting their stems on the diagonal and removing any foliage that will sit below the water line (foliage will contaminate the water and kill the flowers).

Hold the blooms next to the container you will be placing them in to decide on the height, and trim again as necessary.

Start to build the posy: place the thickest stem in the middle for strength. Add another thicker stem, crossed over in the vessel. Keep threading the stems through one another in a criss-cross arrangement: this will help the flowers support themselves (rather than the vessel). Support softer stems, such as tulips, with the centre of the arrangement so they are less likely to flop over. Try to include odd numbers of each flower; one, three or five looks good.

Step back and admire your work. Move any flowers around if they don't fit – let them go where they naturally want to sit and don't force them. Work with the different shapes and heights: for example bring shorter stems to the front and leave taller flowers at the back. Play around and have fun; we're not looking for perfection!

To create a hanging for your posy, make a loop with the florist's wire, then wind it round your receptacle several times. Cover with a complementary ribbon.

Leave on doorsteps or door handles to surprise friends.

To care for your posy

- If any stems start to die, remove them from your arrangement so they don't cause the other flowers to decay.
- Change the arrangement's water every couple of days, trimming the ends of the stems each time.
- To perk up your flowers, add a tiny drop of bleach and pinch of sugar to the water.
- Always keep your blooms away from sunlight, heat or draughts and the fruit bowl – some fruits cause flowers to deteriorate.

PRESSED FLOWERS

This is a particularly nostalgic craft from my childhood. It is easy but so satisfying to make, dry and preserve your floral arrangements – you don't even have to have a flower press: greaseproof paper and a stack of heavy books will do the same job!

YOU WILL NEED
Heavy books
Greaseproof paper
Flower posy

Open a book and place a sheet of greaseproof paper on each page.

Arrange the flowers you want to preserve face down on one of the pieces of greaseproof paper: you could press them in a rough posy arrangement (see page 80) or lay out each stem individually.

Close the book, making sure the other sheet of greaseproof paper completely covers the flowers, and stack several more books on top for 7–10 days.

Remove your flowers once they have fully dried out.

You can now use your pressed flowers for gift tags, cards and any crafts you can think of! I love displaying them in clear clip frames to preserve a beautiful memory of early Summer.

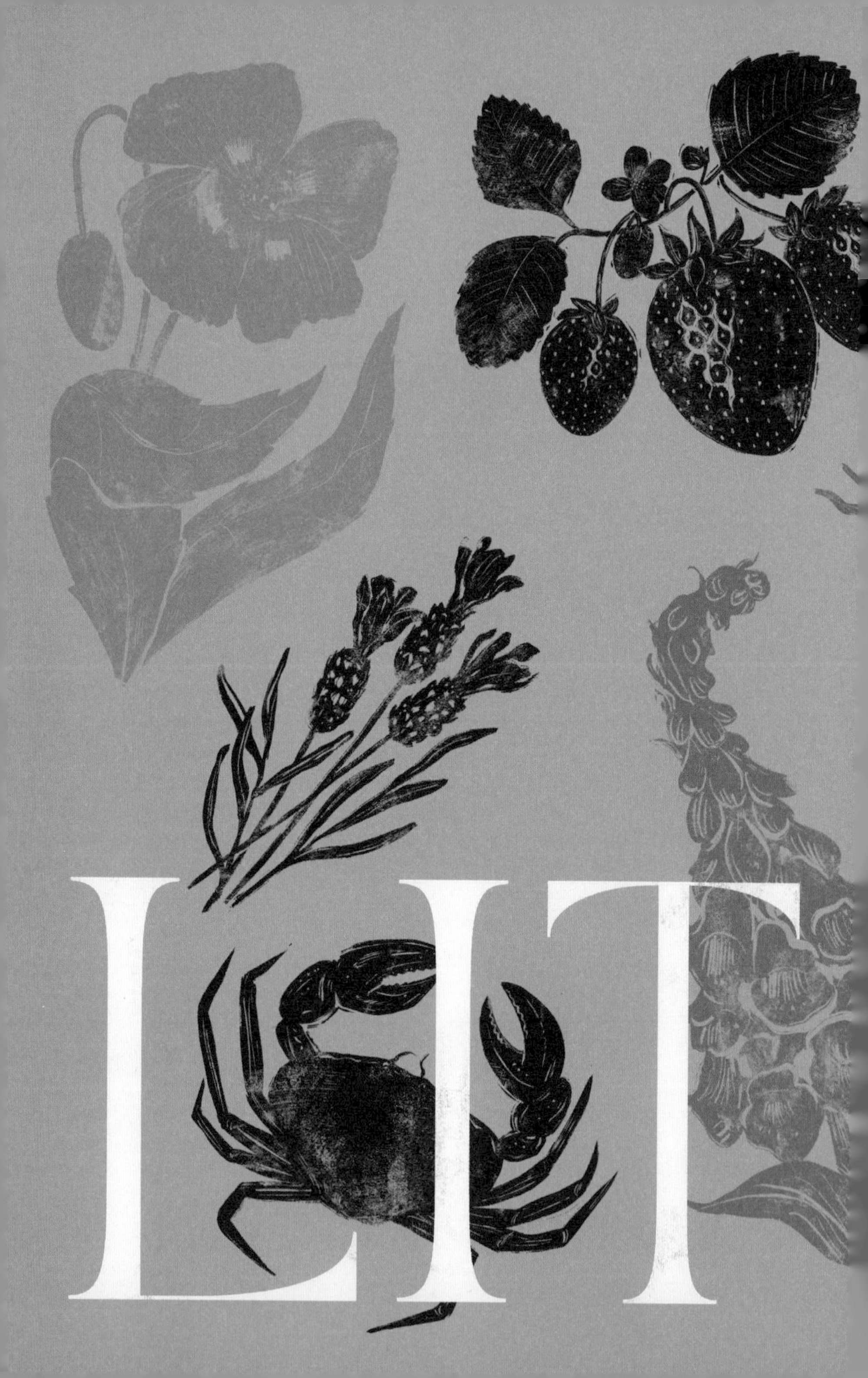
LIT

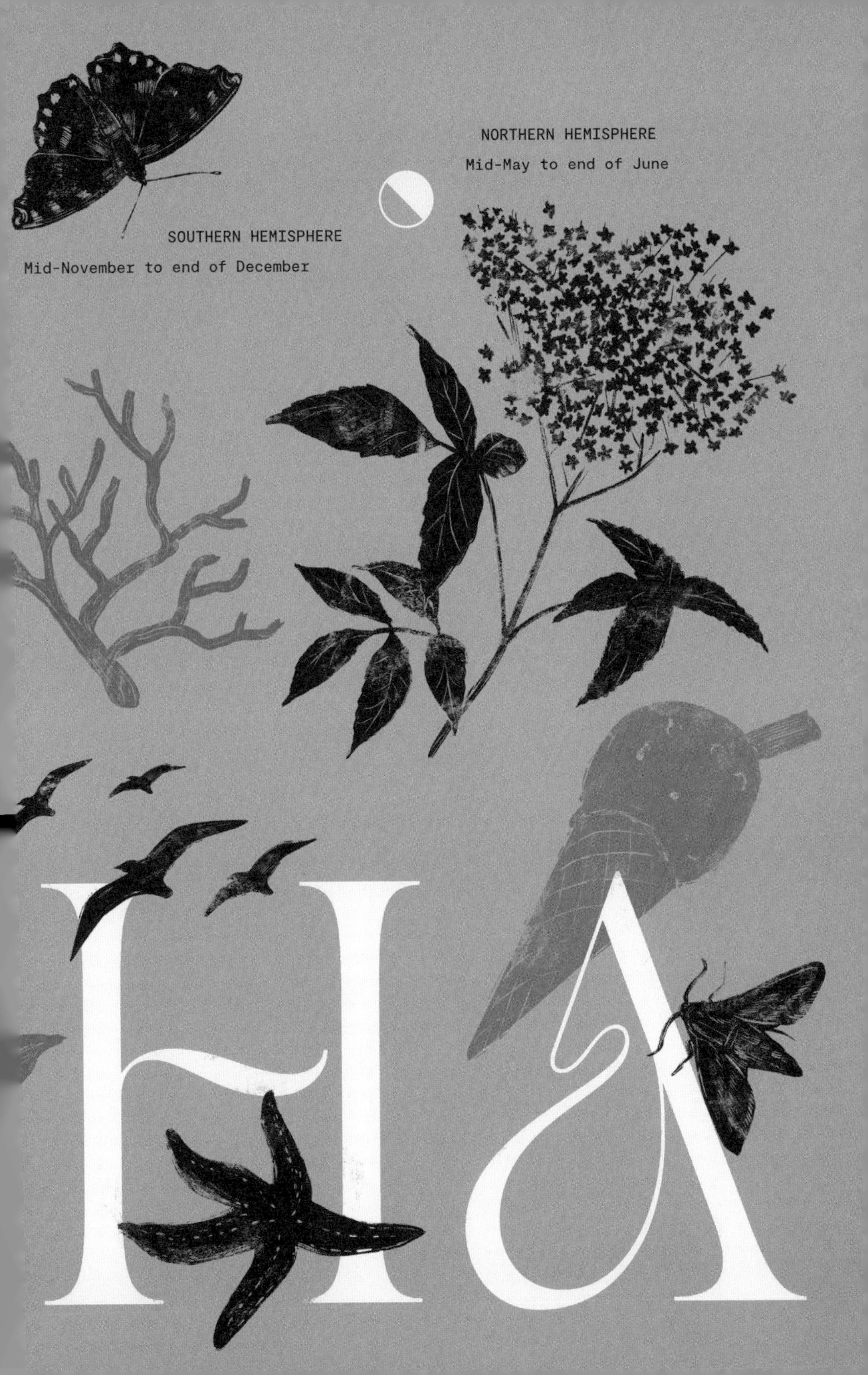
NORTHERN HEMISPHERE
Mid-May to end of June
SOUTHERN HEMISPHERE
Mid-November to end of December

SUMMER SOLSTICE

Litha, the Summer Solstice, marks the longest day of the year: long days and short nights, a landscape full of greenery and optimism. The Summer Solstice has been celebrated for thousands of years across cultures as a time of abundance, fulfilment and joy, and is one of the most important festivals in the Celtic Wheel of the Year. The Celts saw Litha as the second of the Summer holidays after Beltane. It was regarded as a peak – a reminder that the year had turned and that the days would begin getting shorter again – but as well as acknowledging this turning point, Litha was a time for celebration, with bonfires to salute the sun, all-night dancing and merrymaking.

Today Litha usually takes place when the Earth is tilted closest to the sun – a timing that varies slightly year on year, usually between 20 and 22 June. On the days either side of Litha, here in Scotland it feels as though it barely gets dark. We pay for it in Winter – but everything in balance. For now, the light has won. Midsummer marks the height of so much seasonal goodness. It is also a time of anticipation: the anticipation of the holiday season; the anticipation of sunny days and endless evenings; the anticipation of ice cream and sandy toes and carefree times to come.

HIGH SUMMER INVITES ADVENTURE, AND A CHILDISH SENSE OF FREEDOM.

Growing up in rural Fife, my school holidays were largely spent outside. My family didn't tend to go abroad, but with so much on our doorstep there was always something to explore close to home. To me Litha is bike rides along the coastal path in Aberdour, the silhouette of Arthur's Seat and Edinburgh Castle a shimmering mirage beyond the Firth of Forth. Litha is freckles emerging and the potent scent of factor fifty. It's finding wildflowers by the hedgerows and the smell of elderflower. It's sandcastles in St Andrews, with bucket hats and jelly shoes. It's pitching a tent, homemade ice lollies and dancing through the water sprinkler in the garden.

These days, I tend to still spend Litha outdoors to soak up the light of the longest day in nature. My favourite Litha activity is a sunrise or sunset walk up one of Edinburgh's hills, usually Blackford Hill so I can see Arthur's Seat and the castle. Climbing one of the seven hills is a local tradition after school leavers' balls: I climbed Arthur's Seat, aged eighteen, in Converse trainers and a fancy dress. These days, whichever of the seven hills I end up at, I'm usually better equipped with a blanket and basket of treats to enjoy when I get to the top. I always moan about the walk up, but the views across the city are always, always worth it.

The Summer holidays were a time for family celebrations. This always involved me helping Gran set a buffet table for the extended family – the best linen and cutlery saved for celebrations, her favourite sweet peas grown by Granda in small jugs dotted along the table. I still smile at Gran's idea of 'just a salad': a table heaving with the expected lettuce, tomatoes, beetroot, boiled eggs and carrot salads, but also overflowing bowls of crisps, sausage rolls, at least three quiches – and that's before you get to the dessert. You can maybe see why I'm a feeder...

All this being said, as someone who has struggled with their mental health, I'm keenly aware that sometimes this time can be rife with FOMO: fear of missing out. In the darkest days of my twenties, the Summers were often the toughest of all – a time of burnout after long school years, the loss of routine, the feeling that everyone but me was having fun, the loneliness. When you are depressed, it doesn't matter what's happening outside. And even if you're not, Summer can fail to live up to the expectation we Brits so often hopefully imbue it with. A reality of soggy sandwiches, grey days and horizontal rain often put paid to the rose-tinted anticipation of childhood Summers.

But, since I began to tune into seasonal rhythms and traditions more and my mood improved, I've come to embrace both the anticipation and the reality of Summer: the frantic countdown to the holidays and the stillness that follows in all its rainy, sometimes banal, reality. For me, embracing our connections with nature and each other is key. I've learnt that the magic really is in the small moments: the taste of the first Scottish strawberry of the season; a haphazard bunch of flowers grown by someone you love; the green of the landscape after rain; the sound of the tide at the seashore.

Small moments of Summer magic. The Solstice is here.

Seasonal Celebrations at Home

During Litha the whole world seems to be a hive of activity as nature blooms, crops ripen and we reap what we have sown. In recent years, I've embraced the simplest Summer celebrations closer to home.

Pick Your Own

As someone who does not have their own garden but longs to live the good life, visiting a pick-your-own farm gives a dose of escapism. Spending a morning at a fruit farm means you get to spend time in nature and engage all your senses in the activity of fruit picking. Nothing compares to the scent of ripe strawberries picked straight from the plant, or the flavour of a sun-warmed, freshly picked raspberry. Hunt for the biggest, juiciest and ripest fruit and imagine the taste you will savour.

Picking your own fruit means you also get to make something when you get home. Spend the afternoon in the kitchen preparing your pickings: hulling, topping and tailing, chopping. Then the ritual of stirring a pot of bubbling jam, bringing it to a boil, testing for setting point and decanting it into jam jars. A memory of Summer that will taste all the sweeter when opened on a cold Winter day.

Holidays at Home

Growing up, we explored locally rather than going abroad in the holidays: from the beaches of the East Neuk to the galleries and museums of Edinburgh. My simplest adventures were at home, in the garden and along the avenue; joy was in my surroundings and my imagination.

These days I try to capture the essence of simpler times by planning days out close to home. The Summer tourist influx in Edinburgh prompts me to see my city with an outsider's eyes. Visiting historic properties reminds me of my heritage, while walking in natural beauty spots reminds me how lucky I am. Plan a day out in your own hometown and play tourist. You might visit places you've never been, discover things you didn't know or find hidden spots in plain sight. It's amazing how exploring can shift your perspective and reinvigorate a love of where you live.

No-churn Ice Cream

My favourite place to get ice cream treats from is Mary's Milk Bar: a vintage-inspired gelato emporium in the shadow of Edinburgh Castle filled with inventive seasonal flavours. At home – sadly minus ice cream maker – I usually make Nigella Lawson's no-churn ice cream. It is utterly delicious, but I don't always have condensed milk. One day I decided to experiment with something I do always have: custard powder. And my own no-churn ice cream was born:

Make up 200ml custard and chill until firm. Whip 200ml double cream to soft peaks. Remove the custard from the fridge and whisk by hand to remove any lumps. Fold the custard into the whipped cream, along with 50g icing sugar and 1 tablespoon vanilla extract, being careful not to overwhip. Pour into an airtight container and top with greaseproof paper to avoid ice crystals forming. Freeze for several hours, or overnight. Remove the container a little before you want to serve, scoop and enjoy with toppings of your choice.

Rainy Summer Days

Inevitably, at some point it is going to rain and you are going to be disappointed by Summer. As someone who not-so-secretly loves Autumn, I'm always slightly relieved. Growing up, I used to love the sound of the rain drumming on the surface of the pitched roof window in my wee attic bedroom on wet and windy days. I still find the sound of rain incredibly soothing. Rainy days off call for slow kitchen pottering – podding peas or broad beans for instance – and baking with sunshine flavours instead. Perhaps treat yourself to a reading day off and spend an entire afternoon reading a book, cover to cover, to fully immerse yourself in a fictional world. Allow yourself this time and space. When better than a rainy Summer day?

LAVENDER CRÈME BRÛLÉE

Around Litha, the lavender starts to flower and release its summery scent. Lavender farms offer a spectacular sight: field upon field of bright purple flowers swaying in the breeze. You might even be able to pick some yourself, or buy freshly harvested lavender from the farm.

If you want to cook with it, you will need culinary lavender that has not been treated with pesticides; you can source it from local health food stores or find it online. Floral flavours may not be for everyone, but I love to infuse baking with flowers in Summer. Lavender can be made into a floral sugar to be baked into cakes or infused in creams.

SERVES 2

- 275ml double cream
- 100ml semi-skimmed or whole milk
- 1 tbsp dried culinary lavender
- 20g caster sugar
- 3 free-range egg yolks
- 2 tsp demerara sugar, for sprinkling

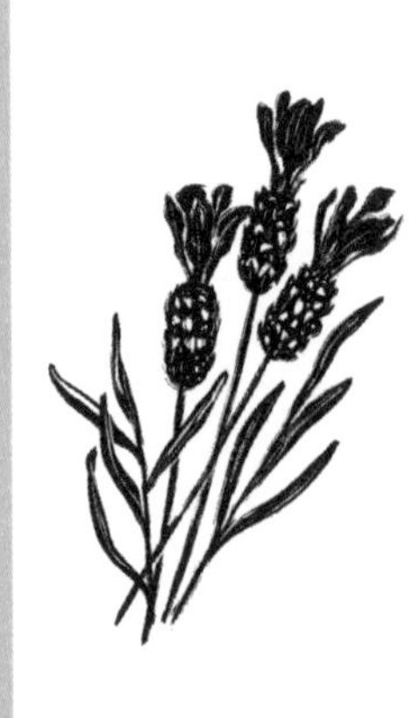

Pre-heat the oven to 160°C/Fan 140°C/Gas Mark 3 and grease two large ramekins.

Heat the cream, milk and lavender in a saucepan over a low heat until just starting to boil. Set aside to infuse for 30 minutes.

Once the time is up, whisk the caster sugar and egg yolks together in a medium-sized bowl.

Bring the cream to just before the boil again, and then strain into a heatproof jug to remove the lavender, before pouring over the egg yolks, stirring the mixture constantly.

Pour this lavender custard into the greased ramekins and place them in a large roasting tin. Pour water around the ramekins (being careful not to splash any into the custard) until halfway up their sides. Cook in the oven for around 15 minutes until set but with a slight wobble.

Remove from the oven and set aside to cool for around 30 minutes, then chill in the fridge until stone cold.

A few hours before you are ready to serve them, pre-heat the grill to a medium–high temperature.

Sprinkle the top of each lavender custard with a teaspoon of demerara sugar, then pop them under the hot grill until melted and golden brown – around 8–10 minutes (keep a close eye on them to make sure they don't burn).

Chill for a few hours and serve.

Note

These are lovely served with the shortbread on page 167: simply replace the pine sugar with standard caster sugar and 1 teaspoon of finely chopped dried culinary lavender.

Summer Solstice Celebration

The Summer Solstice takes place between 20 and 22 June, depending on the year, while the Celts reportedly celebrated Litha on 23 and 24 June. The Summer Solstice is officially the longest day and shortest night of the year, as the Earth is tilted closest to the sun.

Many agricultural societies around the world celebrate the Summer Solstice in some form, worshipping the sun and the abundant daylight it provides. Lots of these celebrations involve an element of magic and the supernatural: in English folklore it was believed that fairies appeared on Midsummer's Eve; and in South America, paper boats were filled with flowers, set on fire and used to send messages to the gods.

Although there are few sources that capture the exact traditions of the ancient Celts in depth, and customs certainly varied, folklore tells us that Litha was a time of celebration and plenty, blessing the crops and land with fire. To mark Midsummer, people would stay up all night on Midsummer's Eve to welcome the sunrise with huge bonfires and merrymaking on hills and in sacred places. As with Beltane, there would be dancing and leaping over the fire for good fortune and to symbolise the light defeating the darkness. Heather torches would be lit and carried to homes and fields to bless them, while the embers of the Midsummer bonfire would be spread on the fields for good luck and a healthy harvest.

The Celts believed that demons and dark magic would be banished by the sunlight, paving the way for months of growth, plenty and good fortune. At the same time, Litha is a reminder of the darkness to come: to quote many a Scottish granny, after Litha the nights will be 'fair drawin' in'. The Celts held the idea of light and dark in balance. Some accounts describe how large wooden wheels were set on fire and rolled down hills into streams, perhaps a symbolic acknowledgement of the waning power of the sun as the Wheel of the Year turned. With growing Christianity, the celebrations became known as St John's Day, celebrating John the Baptist, and dancing and revelry were discouraged.

Oak trees are traditionally associated with Midsummer, as in Celtic mythology the Oak King ruled during Litha. Oaks have long been symbols of fortitude and power, and the trees were often decorated with coloured fabrics. Bonfires were frequently made from oak, and herbs, such as St John's Wort, which was used for luck, would be burnt on the fire or given as gifts alongside birch for protection. Elderflower – which peaks around this time – was meant to ward off witches.

The Summer Solstice was also a holiday of sorts, as it came between sowing and harvesting, meaning those who worked the land had time to slow down during the growing season. For this reason, many weddings took place around this time, the word 'honeymoon' originating from the Honey Moon, the full moon of June, so called because people believed it was the best time to harvest honey.

During Litha, the earth has warmed and nature is at the height of its powers. Taking advantage of the daylight and spending as much time outdoors as possible is essential: creating a wholesome meal with foods that celebrate the light and power of the sun, hosting a family barbecue, creating a beach bonfire and gathering in a circle around it, or climbing a hill and watching the late sunset. Regardless of what you do, Midsummer is a reminder that we are all connected to something bigger. Reflect on the last season and relish your dreams for the season ahead.

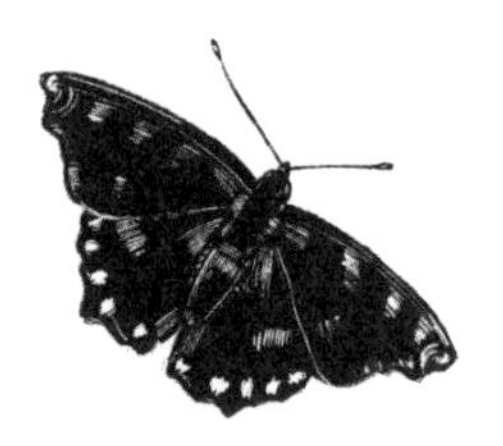

WILDFLOWERS TO FORAGE

Herbs and wildflowers were traditionally foraged at Midsummer to decorate, and for symbolic reasons. Placing flowers under your pillow was meant to inspire your dreams, while lovers would throw flowers over the bonfire, a token of affection.

Elderflower is a short-lived bloom that flowers in hedgerows, woodlands, roads, paths and waste ground. According to folklore, it was said to offer powerful protection and its tiny, creamy-white clusters of umbelliferous flowers certainly look magical. Its scent is the signature scent of Summer for me, and it is a forager's favourite – ideal for infusing cordials or making champagnes or shrubs. It is best harvested in moderation on a warm, sunny day.

Common poppies also start flowering in June; they are surely one of the most distinctive wildflowers due to their bright red petals, which tend to fall off soon after picking them. Their sculptural seed heads are just as beautiful.

The deep-pink–red flowers of red valerian are also distinctive, growing on tall stems in seemingly hostile places such as clifftops and old walls.

It's hard to miss oxeye daisies: they usually grow in swathes along roadsides and next to fields, and have large white petals and yellow centres. They flower from June to September and were colloquially known as 'moon daisies' or 'moonpennies' because of the way their translucent petals glow at dusk.

FLOWER CROWN

Recalling the floral folklore and the celebrations of Litha at Midsummer, making your own flower crown is a fun activity to make at home after foraging for your own wildflowers using the tips on the previous page; perfect for wearing at a Midsummer party. You will need to collect a variety of smaller 'filler' flowers and bigger 'focal' flowers.

YOU WILL NEED

Old cloth or newspaper
Florist's wire
Scissors or secateurs
A big bunch of small and big wildflowers
Ribbon, to decorate (optional)

First, protect your table or work surface by covering it with an old cloth or newspaper.

To weave a base for your flower crown: measure the florist's wire roughly twice around the circumference of your head, then add a little extra to accommodate the flowers. Cut to size.

Bend the cut wire into a circle, winding the wire around itself twice to make a double-layered base.

Prepare your wildflowers to attach to the base by making lots of miniature posies: cut three or five flowers, trim their stems until they are 3–5cm long and wire them together. Group smaller, delicate flowers (for the filler) and larger, statement flowers, so you have a variety of textures. You will need a lot more posies than you think!

Starting with the lighter, more fragile flowers, place a posy onto the base, then attach by wrapping wire around your circlet a few times, and secure it at the back.

Layer another posy on top of the stems of the previous posy to cover the wire. Attach with another piece of wire.

Repeat, adding each posy in the same direction to build volume.

Once you've filled the circumference with the lighter flowers, add the bigger blooms on top to make highlights with the larger flowers.

Don't be precious – the more random and rustic the better. Cover any gaps with filler flowers, hiding the wire inside the flower crown.

Identify the front and tie the ribbon into a bow at the back.

Faff around until you have your desired look, then don with pride!

Tips

- Decide on a palette before you start: simple white and green is lovely or go all out with a multicoloured Midsummer flower crown.
- Make your flower crown just before you want to wear it, as it will start to go limp soon after it's made.
- You could use flowers that can dry out, such as oxeye daisies.

Seasonal Celebrations of Nature

The height of Summer, sunshine and daylight mean abundance and great activity in the natural world. Baby birds are getting ready to fledge – watch from a safe distance as they learn to fly and prepare to leave the nest. If you have a garden, top up your bird bath with water during warm weather (while following current guidance on bird flu, if appropriate).

Dog roses are in full bloom, as is the honeysuckle, both adding a delicious scent to the air and attracting moths and butterflies. The best time to watch them is first thing in the morning as they warm their wings in the sun. You can make a simple feeder to attract butterflies to observe by placing over-ripe fruit, such as bananas, on a plate in the garden. Watch them taste with their feet to assess whether the surface is suitable for them to lay eggs on and feed their young.

The hedgerows and verges fill with thistles, scabious, elderflowers and other wildflowers. Foxgloves are plentiful in woodlands, while fields and verges see numerous poppies, oxeye daisies and buttercups. This is when insects are most abundant: crickets, grasshoppers, daddy-long-legs and bluebottles buzz away in the background. June is the best time to spot wild orchids in the UK, particularly the common spotted variety that are prolific in grassland.

Meadows are a haven for wildlife and promote diversity, particularly of butterflies and bees. Leafcutter bees are busy making nests and you can spot plenty of butterflies, particularly the red peacock butterfly with its distinctive eye-like patterns, the orange and black speckled comma butterfly, the cabbage white and maybe even a red admiral with its red and white markings. During the evenings you can see nocturnal moths, the most exotic-looking being the elephant hawkmoth with green and pink wings or the ermine moth, which actually looks like it is wearing a tiny, spotty, regal cloak!

During warm and dry weather you can spot bats flying at dawn and dusk around woodlands and even in the city, hunting for insects after they emerge from hibernation. In Summer, bats give birth to and raise their pups. Look out for bat watching walks and activities near where you live. As the weather gets warmer, adders and common lizards seek shelter in the shade to stay cool in the south.

At the coast, spot seabirds and their young around the clifftops; the likes of kittiwakes and young guillemots compete for territory. The din you might hear at the seaside is the sound of hungry gull chicks in their clifftop colonies. You can still spot many birds feeding their fledglings, particularly wagtails in the trees and stonechats on the moors. Snow white Arctic terns with their black caps arrive in their hundreds of thousands all the way from Antarctica. Beware their territorial instincts – particularly their bright beaks, which are razor sharp.

This is a great time to go rock pooling. Check when low tide is, and make sure you wear wellies or sturdy shoes with good grip. Take a book, such as an *Observer's Book* or similar, to identify your finds, plus maybe a camera for photos or a sketchpad to draw any wildlife you see. Move carefully so you don't disturb anything (or slip on seaweed, abundant around Litha) and avoid standing in the rockpools. Wildlife is most interesting observed in its natural habitat, especially if you check beneath rocks and in corners. Look out for crabs, starfish, limpets and snails and observe them – but remember not to handle the wildlife.

Wildflowers can flourish at the seashore too, particularly thrift, which loves salty sea air. Its pink, pompom-like flowers are in bloom in early Summer, forming a seemingly incongruous display of pink and green against the cliffs. By Midsummer, fish in rivers begin their Summer run, with salmon and trout plentiful and increasing in numbers as Summer continues. Spot them after rain when rivers are fuller, which encourages more underwater activity.

Seaweed

I was lucky enough to grow up in a wee seaside village on the Fife coast, so the sea is in my soul. It is where I go to feel calm in any season, even adoring the barren, stormy beaches of Winter, but there is something about the magic of the seaside in Summer I can't resist. Its rhythmic ebb and flow never fails to ground me and I feel most at home on the beach.

It's a cliché, but the vast openness of the sea, its infinite nature, shrinks my problems – and myself in comparison. Perhaps it's the multi-sensory experience it evokes – the scent of salt water you can almost taste, the din of the waves and the regular rhythm of their movement.

I am biased, but the east coast is home to some of my favourite beaches; their shores punctuate many of my happiest memories. From the sandy beaches of East Lothian, where regular trips to accessible and beautiful North Berwick kept me grounded on dark days; to the three beaches of St Andrews, where I remember family days and, later, university nights; and to the rugged coast of Aberdeenshire where I visited my partner during his PhD. Each has a place in my story, has helped and healed me.

But I will always come back to the beaches of my home, Aberdour: Silver Sands and Black Sands. These small but perfectly formed sandy bays look out over the Firth of Forth to Edinburgh, and past Inchcolm Island and its famous abbey. Passing behind is my beloved Fife Coastal Path, with beautiful woodland walks, and memories of spotting boats in the harbour and crossing the 'trip trap' bridge in Summer.

When I was wee, I would collect shells on every beach visit, but these days I'm more interested in seeing the plant life, spotting types of seaweed, sketching, photographing or preserving my finds.

Seaweed is often overlooked; I only really started to appreciate the different shapes and varieties when I found out that you can press and preserve it, and began to admire the range of organic textures, colours and creative potential this natural material provides.

Collecting Seaweed

There are thousands of species of seaweed, which are usually grouped into red, green and brown. They grow on seashores and the bottom of the sea. Seaweed is easy to find on the shore as it needs light to photosynthesise and provide the plant with its energy. The intertidal zone (the area above water level at low tide but underwater at high tide) is the best place to find it – look for it in rocky areas, where it can easily attach.

Incidentally, many seaweeds are edible (and there are thankfully no poisonous seaweeds on the British coast) and have been foraged as food for hundreds of years. Regardless of whether you plan on eating them or not, make sure to collect your specimens away from sources of pollution (download the Safer Seas Service app to check how clean the water is) and steer clear of anything that smells or is rotting. It goes without saying that you should keep an eye on the tides, which change quickly, and try to go collecting with a friend if you can – or at least let someone know where you are and when to expect to hear from you.

When collecting seaweed to press, find smaller pieces to work with – no bigger than a piece of A4 paper. Make sure no wildlife is clinging to your seaweed as you shouldn't disturb it. Never pull seaweed off rocks, as this would cause damage to this important ecosystem; make sure you have the landowner's permission; and cut only up to the top third of growth. If you are using the seaweed for just crafting, you can use free floating seaweed, which you can remove without the landowner's permission. Look for pieces at low tide that have naturally washed up, either on the beach or floating in rockpools or shallow water.

You never know what you're going to find: observe the different colours in different seasons, temperatures and light levels. Collecting seaweed after a storm can provide a greater range of interesting specimens, thrown up from the depths below. Here are ten different types of seaweed to look out for on your next beach trip:

RED

Purple laver

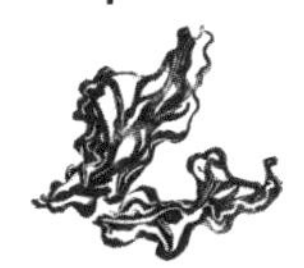

This seaweed has thin, purple-brown fronds and is commonly found at the top of rocky beaches. It is used in salty Welsh laver bread.

Coral weed

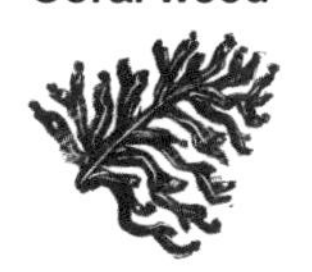

Another smaller seaweed, which is pink or purple (depending on where it is found) and has rigid fronds creating a feathery appearance. It is common in rockpools.

Carageen/Irish moss

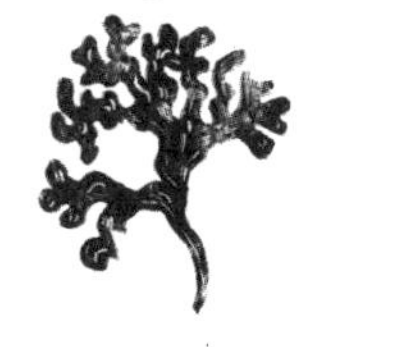

This has flat, long fronds and is a distinctive dark purple. It is edible and is often used as a thickener in commercial sauces.

GREEN

Bladderwrack

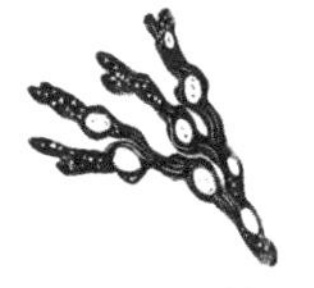

The air 'bladders' on this olive-green seaweed are the source of its name. It can usually be found in the middle of the shore.

Gut weed/grass kelp

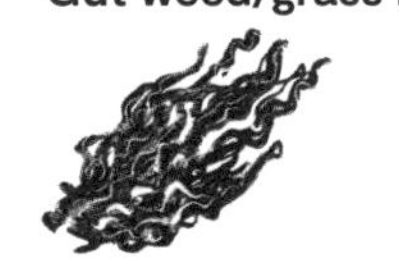

A common, bright-green seaweed with tubular fronds that appear grass-like; air bubbles sometimes trap in them, giving it the look of an intestine.

Sea lettuce

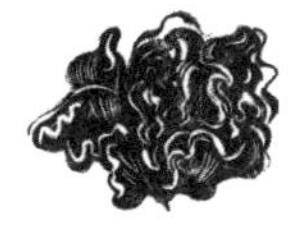

This is a small green seaweed that is – you guessed it – shaped like a lettuce. It tends to grow on rocks on the mid-shore. It is edible: dehydrated, it has a strong umami flavour.

BROWN

Channelled wrack

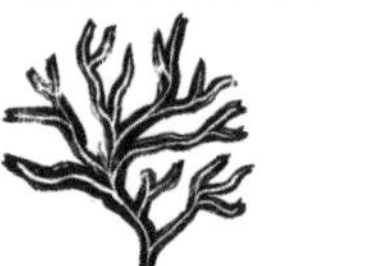

A very common yellowish-brown seaweed with curled, medium-sized fronds that create a channel shape. It is usually found at the top of the shore.

Pepper dulse

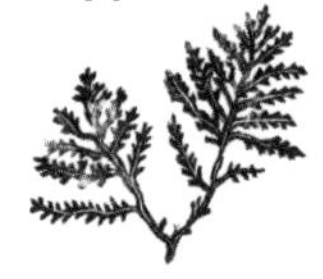

This small reddish-brown species has a distinctive flattened fern shape. You might have heard dulse being referred to as 'truffle of the sea' when used in cuisine.

Oarweed

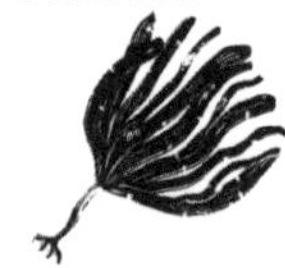

Revealed at low tide, this common seaweed has glossy, greenish-brown fronds that split into two and reach up to two metres long.

Sugar kelp

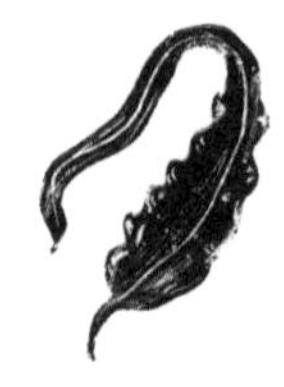

Another common brown seaweed that has very long fronds with a frilly edge, found in deep pools and after storms. It is sometimes used in cooking as a sugar substitute.

PRESSING SEAWEED

Pressing seaweed is a simple way to preserve your specimens: indeed, it was once a popular pastime of Victorian women, Queen Victoria herself being said to possess an album of pressed seaweed. When pressing your finds the main ingredient is time, as it can take a while to dry out, but it is a great slow Summer project that you can then use in lots of different ways (see below). Seaweed creates a beautiful palette of olive greens, rich plums and surprising pinks.

YOU WILL NEED

Seaweed specimens
5cm-deep tray
1 sheet of thick paper, e.g. watercolour paper (any size to fit your tray)
Thin paint brush
Tea towel
Kitchen paper
Greaseproof paper
Scrap cardboard or newspaper
Large flower press or stack of heavy books

Thoroughly rinse the seaweed to remove any sand or dirt.

Half fill the tray with water and place the thick paper on the bottom.

Arrange the seaweed over the paper, using the paint brush to help if you need to encourage it into place: bits might float to the surface, but you can still arrange your desired pattern.

Gently reach underneath the paper and lift it out, keeping it as flat as you can. Place it on top of the tea towel.

Carefully dry the paper with kitchen paper, dabbing it gently. Rearrange the seaweed if you need to.

Cover the surface of the paper and specimens with more kitchen paper, then a layer of greaseproof paper.

Place the scrap card or newspaper on top, then place your paper, cardboard and all, inside a flower press or underneath a stack of heavy books.

Each day, check on it and change the greaseproof paper and kitchen paper closest to the specimens.

Repeat until the seaweed has completely dried out. Smaller pieces will dry out quickly, but larger samples might take a week or more.

When dried, carefully remove the seaweed from the paper and use as desired.

What to make with your pressed seaweed

- Stick it onto a greetings card using glue, or use the seaweed shapes to decorate gift tags.
- Frame your best pressed samples and admire them. Simple clear clip frames allow the specimen to take centre stage.
- For bigger pieces, cut out shapes freehand or with a stamper and use them as confetti or to decorate all manner of items.

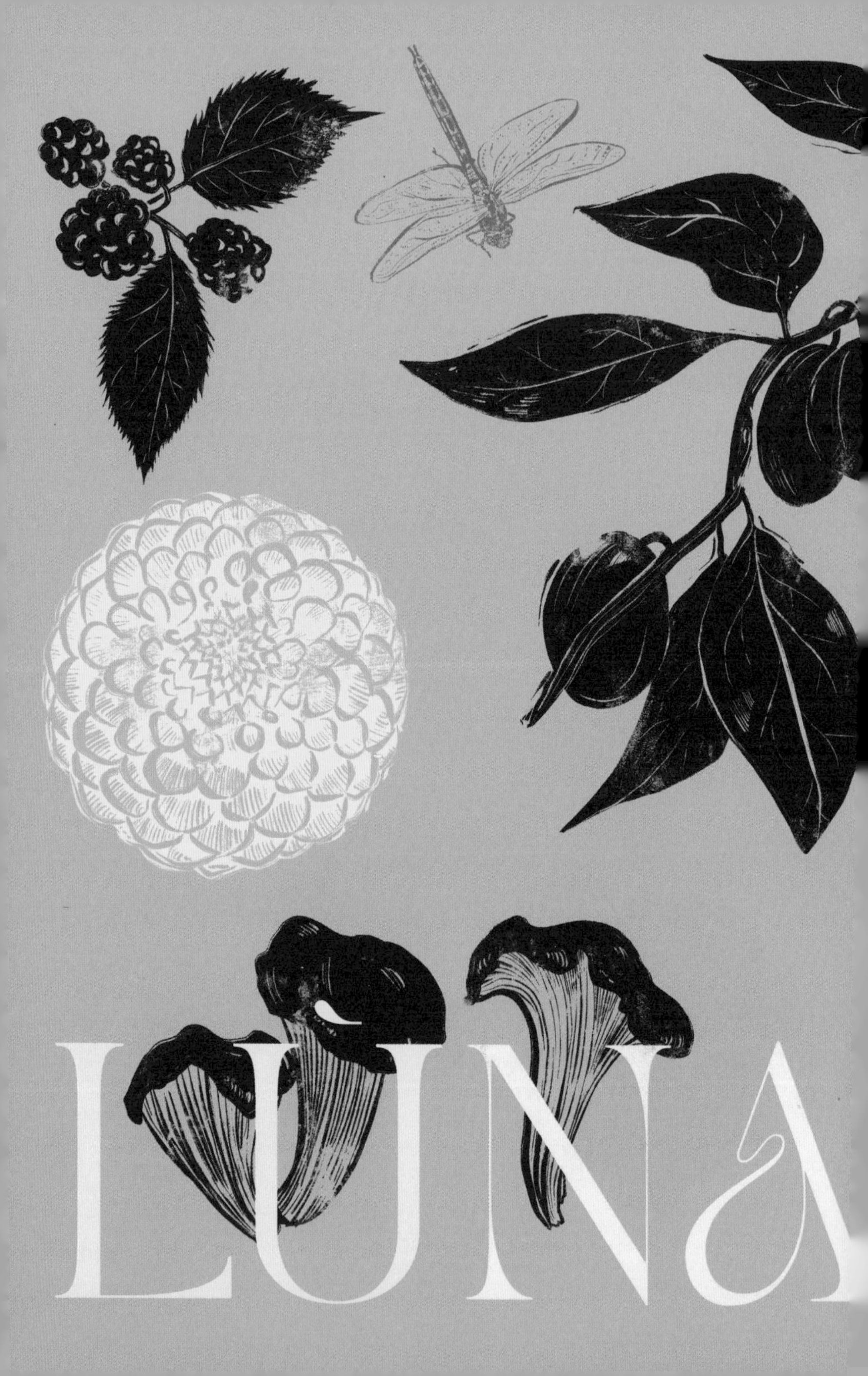
LUNA

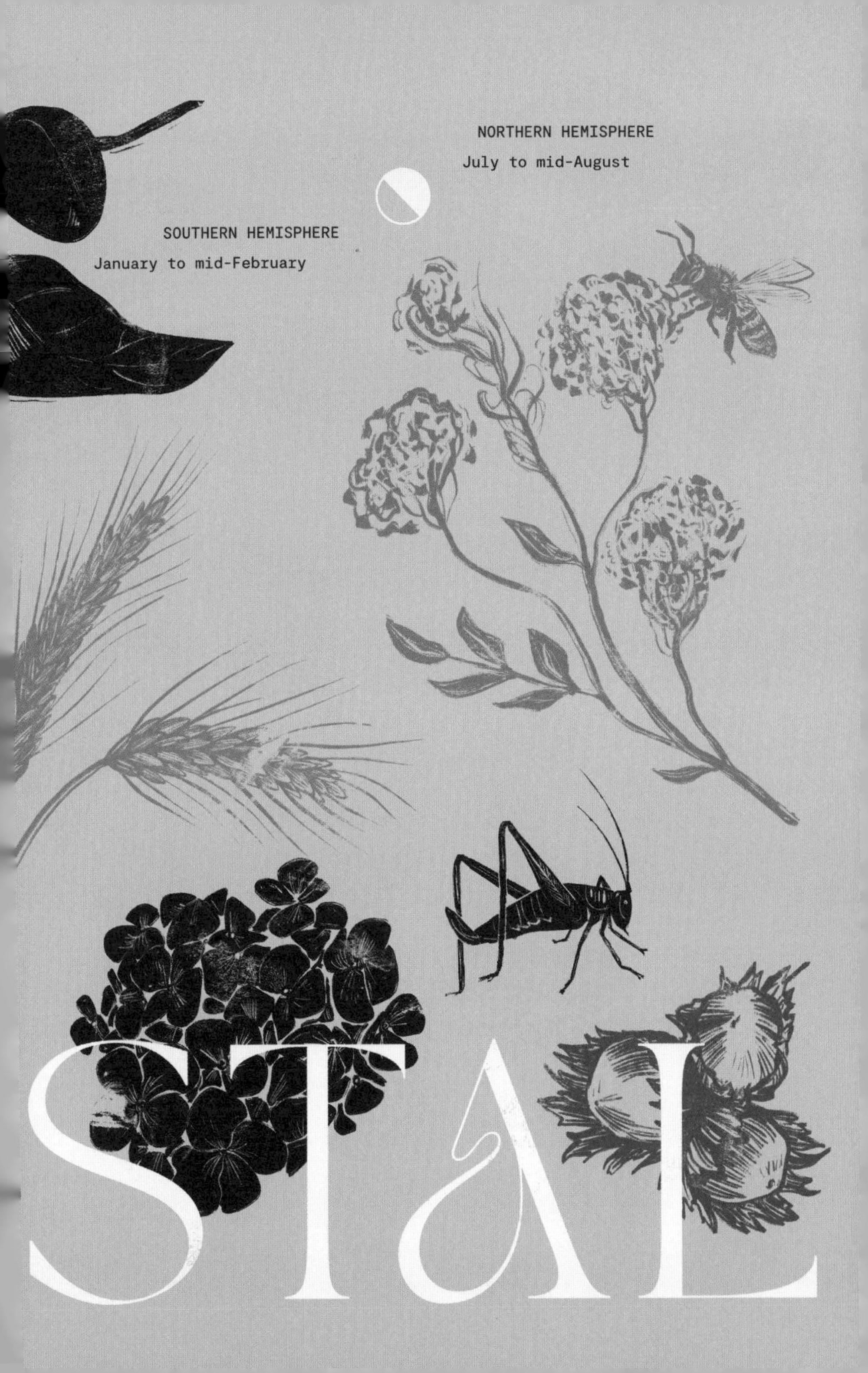
NORTHERN HEMISPHERE
July to mid-August
SOUTHERN HEMISPHERE
January to mid-February
STAL

HARVEST

The countryside glows golden as Summer's light ripens the grains and swells the fruit and vegetables ready for harvesting. Lùnastal (pronounced 'LOO-nas-til') on 1 August is the start of the harvest season, known as Lammas in the Christian calendar, and a time to truly celebrate abundance.

This six-week period leading up to and around Lùnastal marks many seasonal changes, from the height of Summer to early Autumn and all its joys: dahlias begin to bloom, the sunshine is golden, fields of barley and wheat ripen, and orchard fruits mature on the trees. A seasonal shift is in the air as the Celtic Wheel of the Year turns; we become all too aware of Summer's fleeting nature as the nights creep ever so slightly shorter and nature begins to sigh and slow.

The holiday period offers a chance to celebrate Summer and its abundant seasonal food and flowers. Here in Scotland, we break at the end of June for the Summer holidays, and the school year begins again in August, so the period up to and around Lùnastal takes us from Summer freedom to back-to-school feeling. Returning to school was a time of contradictions for me, often getting the best of the late sunny weather when I was stuck in my school kilt, which gave me a simultaneous sadness at saying goodbye to Summer and excitement for the fresh start of the Autumn term.

Lùnastal also meant the last few weekend treats, escapes and celebrations. Several family birthdays gave us a good reason to set the table and bake a cake, usually a pavlova – any flavour; you choose! – at my brother's request, and a chocolate cake at Granda's. There was always some sort of traditional crafting with Mum and Gran at the kitchen table too: a dress or top for the last Summer outings; lavender bags made with fabric from the scraps box and pouches of dried flowers; or pressing blooms from the last of Summer's adventures between the pages of a textbook, to be forgotten about and rediscovered with delight in many months.

Lùnastal to me is blackberries: Dad, Granda and I were all berry fiends and I can still taste Gran's traditional 'plate cake', filled with blackberries picked from the garden between layers of crisp pastry, eaten warm from the oven and covered in cream. I still make a version of the same cake that takes me straight back to childhood.

We're officially in the latter half of the year now.

THE EARTH KEEPS TURNING AND THE FIRST FLICKERS OF AUTUMN CAN BE INCREASINGLY SPOTTED.

From the changing light in the evenings and the gradual golden transformation of the countryside to the very first yellow leaves, fading flowers and drying seed heads. A whisper of the season to come.

Seasonal Celebrations at Home

At home and close to home there are so many transitional moments to savour. The flower world still blooms, early Summer's varieties giving way to late Summer showstoppers, such as dahlias, rudbeckias and hydrangeas. Arrangements embody this time of year's abundance, whether you have your own cutting patch or source them from a local flower farm. Ripening golden fields seem to beckon; pack a picnic and enjoy it by a meadow – you can find beautiful public spaces being rewilded with fields of wildflowers and swaying grasses. Bake fresh bread from locally milled flour and harvest seasonal fruit and vegetables to enjoy or preserve for the colder months. Escape for a while to refresh your senses, and begin some gentle preparation for the seasons ahead, as we enter the second half of the Wheel of the Year.

Back to Basics

Some days I just want to pack it all in and move to a cabin in the woods, or a hut in the hills, be totally self-sufficient and throw my phone in a loch. This happens when I need a break and to truly switch off with a change of scene, which is usually around now! And it seems I'm not the only one: in recent years, probably exacerbated by the pandemic, remote escapes – spaces that allow you to make yourself at home off-grid, for a little while at least – have been popping up more prolifically.

Exhausted after teaching through the pandemic, my partner and I each packed a backpack with just the essentials and drove to Inverlonan in the Highlands to a secret wilderness where we stayed at Beatha (Bay-ah) Bothy, looking out over the shores of Loch Nell and surrounded by ancient oak trees. The cabins are beautifully designed with luxurious finishes but are literally in the middle of nowhere – accessed only on foot or by boat

– and have no running hot water, flushing toilet or mains shower. It was bliss. Firing up the stove to heat our water and the snail's pace everything took was so refreshing. We were forced to completely slow down; small daily acts like making a cup of coffee, showering or cooking took up a surprisingly substantial amount of the day. We foraged for hazelnuts by the loch, cooked over the open fire and simply watched the scenery, spotting red squirrels, deer and Highland cows. Returning home, I saw everything with fresh eyes: off-grid stays can help put things into perspective by reminding you that the most simple things are the most satisfying, and the daily acts that we take for granted can be moments of everyday magic.

Back-to-School Feeling

As August arrives, I begin to feel the seasonal shift as my thoughts turn towards preparing for the new school year. The academic calendar is so deeply engrained in me now that it's practically part of my inner clock. And I'm sure I'm not the only one – anyone still in education, with children or who works in an academic setting no doubt has that 'back-to-school feeling' around Lùnastal. You don't need new shoes and a pencil case to embody this feeling: it can come from within as you reflect on the first half of the year and plan for what's ahead.

This is a time of anticipation and anxiety, perhaps maybe even dread for some of us, surrounding the season ahead and the knowledge of coming darkness, but there's no denying it has the feeling of a fresh start, too; if we try to welcome in this positivity, we can make it work in our favour. Affirmations are something I did as a teen and remind myself to do from time to time. Write them out by hand with a beautiful pen and decorate them. Place them next to a mirror in your bedroom or next to your bedside table as an encouraging reminder. If this makes you feel too self-conscious, perhaps write down in your journal a key word that you want to feel or embody for the season ahead, so you can remind yourself when you need. Look back at old notebooks or photographs, or talk to a friend; and remember how far you have come and how much you have achieved. Worry can be productive too: I always find that taking practical, positive action around something I've been worrying about helps me to feel prepared for the coming months – whether that's a new planner, ticking off some boring life admin or sorting my calendar. I always feel better for it.

Lùnastal Foraging

Warmer weather sees a huge array of foraging potential in the natural world. The first chanterelles begin to appear in woodlands. Their distinctive gold colour, wavy, trumpet shape and stone fruit scent make them one of the easier mushrooms to identify ('false chanterelles' are the same colour but have a traditional mushroom shape and smell). Make sure you check with a trusted source – such as a guidebook or local foraging expert – before eating them; look online for courses near you. When you get home, wash your chanterelles and gently cook them in a little butter, perhaps with thyme or rosemary if you fancy it, then toss through pasta or risottos or serve simply on sourdough toast with a poached egg.

The tall, upright, white frothy flower clusters of meadowsweet are in full bloom along damp verges and roadsides. You can snip a handful of flowers, wrap them in a muslin and use it to infuse in cordials and jams. Meadowsweet has a wonderful almond-like flavour that goes beautifully with Summer fruits such as strawberries and raspberries, which you might just find wild as well. They're like miniature versions of the well-known fruits; their flavour is concentrated and sweet, in a whole other league to their cultivated counterparts. Blaeberries – or bilberries if you are in England – also ripen from July. This cousin of the blueberry grows in surprising places, including heaths and moorland. It has smaller berries, but their flavour is more intense and aromatic, and they will stain your fingers a deep purple. Be sure to pick any of these berries above waist (and dog wee) height, ensure you get a positive identification online or in a foraging handbook and rinse before eating. It'll take a while to forage enough to bake with or preserve, but I think this is a flavour you want to experience in a pure and unadulterated way. Fresh and sun-warmed, they taste of late Summer.

Dried Hydrangeas

As the Summer gardens reach their peak, thoughts turn to preserving flowers. In our old family home, my parents had the most beautiful hydrangea plant that, even when left to its own devices, created pompom flowers as big as your head in shades from cornflour blue to deep purple. I first experimented with drying them when my parents were selling their house in Fife, and I was desperate to hold onto their late Summer beauty. Hardier stems such as hydrangeas are good to start with when drying flowers, as they tend to work beautifully with very little effort.

I always pre-arrange my stems, as they can be quite brittle to handle once dried and therefore difficult to manipulate and arrange effectively. Think about the different heights and spread of colours and textures that will work in your dried arrangement. It will change but this gives you a rough idea of how the dried blooms will look. Then simply leave them in the jar with a tiny amount of water in a totally dark room. Too much water and the stems will mould, too little and they dry too quickly and become shrivelled – so it may take a little trial and error, depending on the variety of your plant and the environment it is in. Another technique is simply to leave them to almost completely dry on the plant, then cut them and bringing them indoors to fully dry. Once your hydrangeas have dried, you can use them as desired: to decorate a late Summer wreath or make a garland from groups of two dried hydrangea hemispheres wired together and attached to twine.

GREENGAGE CRUMBLE LOAF CAKE

The first orchard fruits are ripening and ready for the eating. Plums are my favourite: my grandparents had a Victoria plum tree, and the plums' sharp sweetness reminds me of early Autumn days at their house, where we would eat them fresh from the tree. Greengages are a smaller, slightly sweeter type of plum with a short season – they are delicious eaten raw or baked into a cake such as this one. Like plums, greengages pair well with almonds. This greengage crumble loaf cake can be adapted with any plums or stone fruit combining my two favourite desserts: crumble and cake.

SERVES 8–10

For the topping
- 20g plain flour
- 20g ground almonds
- 20g demerara sugar
- 20g butter
- 2 greengages (or one medium-sized plum), thinly sliced
- 1 tbsp flaked almonds

For the loaf cake
- 180g butter
- 180g light soft brown sugar
- 3 large free-range eggs
- 150g self-raising flour
- 30g ground almonds
- 3 tbsp milk
- 1½ tsp almond extract
- 150g greengages or plums, chopped into chunks

Pre-heat the oven to 180°C/Fan 160°C/Gas Mark 4 and grease and line a 450g loaf tin.

First, prepare your crumble topping. In a bowl, mix together the flour, ground almonds and demerara sugar, then lightly rub in the butter with the tips of your fingers until the mixture looks like breadcrumbs. Set aside.

Then, start on the loaf cake. With a wooden spoon in a bowl or in a stand mixer with the paddle attachment, cream the butter and soft brown sugar until light and very fluffy.

Add one egg to the mixture and beat it in, then add roughly a third of the flour and beat it in too. Repeat with the remaining eggs and flour, beating briefly between additions. Fold in the ground almonds.

Add the milk and almond extract, folding it in lightly.

Fold through the chopped greengages.

Pour the mixture into the prepared loaf tin and level the surface with a spatula.

Arrange the two additional, thinly sliced greengages on top of the cake mixture.

Sprinkle with the crumble topping, followed by the flaked almonds.

Bake for 45–50 minutes or until golden and a skewer inserted in the middle comes out clean. If the crumble starts to become too golden brown, cover the cake with foil for the remainder of the bake time.

Leave to cool in the tin for a few minutes, then remove and cool completely on a wire rack.

HOST A HARVEST FESTIVAL AT HOME

When I was growing up, Lùnastal celebrations were some of the last before the end of the Summer and before the school year began again. They were times to spend with family and look back on the past Summer, to enjoy nature and to share and eat good food.

According to folklore, Lùnastal marks the beginning of the harvest seasons in the Celtic Wheel of the Year and is technically the start of Autumn. It is a celebration of the first Autumn fruits: a time of plenty, as fruit, vegetables and grains are ripe and ready for picking, eating and preserving.

Granda worked in farming, at an auctioneer, and referred to this time onwards as the 'back end of the year': it was certainly a time when deals were done, livestock bought and sold and celebrations had before the harder months to come.

The festival of Lùnastal in Scotland, Lughnasadh in Ireland, was originally thought to occur around the phases of the moon, but the date has been simplified to the first of the month in the modern calendar – and arguably Christianised to coincide with Lammas Day. As with some other celebrations in the Celtic Wheel, sadly much of the history of Lùnastal has been lost in Scotland due to the powerful Kirk, which disapproved of its Pagan origins and discouraged the festival.

What we do know from that time is that Lùnastal maintained the elements of the other festivals in the Celtic Wheel – mainly gatherings and feasting – with the emphasis on harvest sharing closer to home. 'Handfastings' often occurred at this time, partners trialling a year of marriage before deciding whether to commit to one another forever. Smaller hilltop fairs and commercial activities often occurred locally, with the lighting of bonfires, games and dancing.

Lùnastal is a time of conclusion, completion and accomplishment as we move into the darker half of the year, saying goodbye to the warmer weather as the days keep getting shorter. Historically, this would lead to a looming sense of change in the air and a desire for protection as the community entered the darker months. Cows were brought in from pasture at this time, their milk made into cheese, which was meant to bring good luck (as it did not last long). This would also be the end of the fishing season, after which everyone would help with harvesting grain for Winter. Flowers were used to decorate, and grain-based foods were made with the fresh harvest – such as bannocks or porridge – served alongside freshly harvested fruit and vegetables.

Today, Lùnastal coincides with the start of the Edinburgh Fringe, and the Edinburgh International Festival just a few days after that; it is the zenith of the creative calendar here in Scotland. In fact, many festivals take place in the capital during August, including my long-time love, the Edinburgh International Book Festival (now with its new home on Lauriston Place). The city's population more than doubles in size with all the tourists arriving in Edinburgh to see shows and entertainers, or just to soak up the atmosphere. Pubs are given a temporary late licence (some until 5 a.m., long past my bedtime) and there is a feeling of creative possibility in the air.

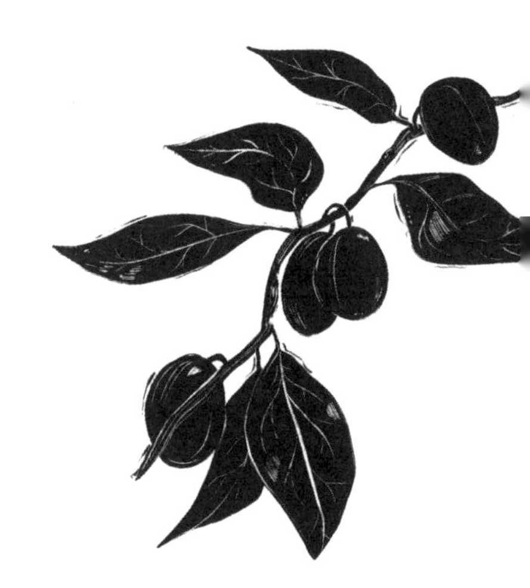

NAPKIN RINGS

Hosting a harvest celebration at home is a way to honour the seasonal shift, to share its spoils and memories before the arrival of Autumn proper. I like to set the table with rustic, faded linens, seasonal dahlias, sheaves of dried wheat or corn, and decorative dried corn cobs. You can get these from local florists, and as they are dried, they can be stored and used again and again. Corn can be woven into wreaths or plaited into dolls, as the tradition goes (often a sign of affection and good luck for the farm), but for a contemporary take I weave mine into decorative napkin rings.

YOU WILL NEED (PER NAPKIN RING)

3 ears of wheat, straws intact, dampened if brittle
Florist's wire
Scissors
Dried flowers (such as poppy seed heads or Astrantia)
Ribbon

Wind florist's wire around the three straws just underneath the ears of wheat to tie them together. Twist to secure.

Plait the straws together: cross the right straw over the middle straw, then the left straw over the new middle straw. Repeat, keeping going until you reach the end.

Bring the end of the plait around to the wire to make a ring. Remove the wire, position the end of the plait so that it is behind the ears of wheat, then wire into place again.

Thread a napkin through so the napkin ring holds its shape as it dries out.

Once it has dried out after a couple of days, wire some dried flowers on top of the ears of wheat, if you like, and finish with a ribbon, tied in a bow.

SUMMER MEMORY BANK

Before moving into the next season, I like to reminisce over the best of the season just gone with this memory bank. You can do this at the end of Summer, or remember to add to it as you go through the season. It gives you something to look back on in the cold, dark months ahead. You can make your jar look pretty, but you don't have to.

This is not just a fun and simple way to preserve memories – recording the small moments you might forget in the hubbub of day-to-day life – there is actually positive brain science behind it. Ronnie, my NHS therapist, was a compassionate man but not a sentimental one (I thought), so I was surprised when he suggested noting memories in this way. Less romantically, he called it 'positive data logging'. By recording small moments when you feel happy and free, you store up a bank of good things you can revisit on darker days: a reminder that there is light in the world. I know that sometimes even this joy can be hard to find. I have been there, trust me, and if you're there right now, I am sending you the biggest hug and oodles of understanding. You are not the only one.

Ronnie, this one's for you.

YOU WILL NEED

- Pieces of coloured paper, cut into strips
- Pretty pens, for writing
- 1-litre Kilner jar
- Polaroids or other printed photographs (small snapshots are good, you can write on the back of them)
- Anything else that evokes a happy memory (optional)

This is a fun activity to do with your family or the special people in your life, or you could do it on your own.

Write a fun Summer memory on a small strip of paper. Focus on a small thing rather than a big thing, so rather than 'Our holiday to Disneyland' (I wish!), break it down to 'the moment I found out we were going on holiday' or 'the feeling of my own bed when I got home from holiday' (you can tell everything you need to know about me from that last one).

Write the date – and your name on the back if you're sharing – and put it into the jar, along with a photo, if you have one – or you could write the memory on the back.

Keep going until you fill up the jar – adding anything else that evokes a happy memory, if you like. You will be surprised how quickly it fills, focusing on the wee things rather than the big ones.

Tip

If you are struggling to find the joy, then I urge you to try making your own. Get up five minutes early to make time for a cup of tea in your favourite mug. Set aside time to make one of the crafts in this book. Treat yourself to your favourite chocolate bar. Read for a while. Banish your phone before bedtime.

SUMMER MEMORY DISPLAY

I have always been a collector. Ever since I was a child, I've been bringing home mementos from walks and days out in nature: feathers, special stones, pretty pine cones and mesmerising shells. Mum has, proudly, kept many of these treasures and I love her for nurturing and valuing that wide-eyed wonder in me.

Nowadays, I try to use my seasonal magpie instinct to my advantage to decorate and create displays. I thrifted a vintage printer's tray at our local salvage yard – the kind that's a flat wooden tray of regularly spaced squares or rectangles with space not much bigger than fits a metal letter from a printing press, maybe with a few bigger holes. They aren't particularly practical as drawers any more, but they are great for making displays and storing small objects. I suppose this is another, more visual, way of recording memories like in the previous craft – and again, it is so simple it barely needs instructions.

YOU WILL NEED

- A receptacle (printer's tray, small shelves, crate or similar)
- Cleaning cloth
- Paint brush
- A collection of souvenirs from your Summer travels or nature finds
- Glue dots or washi tape

Clean your receptacle with the cloth, using the paint brush to get into any stubborn corners. Leave it to thoroughly dry out.

Arrange your objects in the tray in a pleasing way. You could tell a story by arranging the objects in chronological order, or you could group natural objects and others, or arrange by colour... It's up to you.

Once you are happy with the positioning, stick your objects into place – either using a tiny dot of glue if you want to keep the fixing hidden, or using washi tape if you want to make it a feature.

Step back and admire your handiwork. Hang your tray on a wall or prop it up on a table or drawers.

Let the display evolve over time by adding new finds or taking away pieces of nature that look a little tired and replacing them with new ones. Dust your display carefully once in a while, using this mindful activity to reconnect with your finds and enjoy reliving the memories.

Seasonal Celebrations of Nature

In July and August here in the UK, it feels like all of nature is alive. The fields buzz with activity and the hedgerows are abundant following hot days, sunshine and Summer showers. Plenty of wildlife offspring are readying for the big wide world. Stealthy stoats are tricky to spot but you might see their young, practising pouncing. Fox kits (babies) can be spotted in urban areas. Otter cubs are born during the Summer months and – if you're lucky – you might spot females hunting during the day to feed their young, or even cubs exploring later in Summer. Hedgehogs also have broods over summertime, and by the end of the season hoglets become more independent, hunting in gardens to store up food before hibernation – best spotted at dusk.

Golden fields of crops begin to be harvested. The hum of crickets and grasshoppers can still be heard, the former more commonly in the south of the UK. In the meadows and on verges, there is plenty of nectar for busy bees and butterflies: the blue butterfly, with its spectacular ice blue and brown colouring, can be seen in some parts of the UK.

In the hills and on the moors, heather begins to flower, creating a spectacular pinky-purple carpet as far as the eye can see. The most vivid is bell heather, which is practically magenta and can be found in drier areas. Heather blooms into Autumn, creating a feast for buzzing bees. When walking near heather, wear sturdy footwear and be mindful of disturbing hiding birds and animals.

In ponds, frogs, toads and newts can be spotted, as can dragonflies. If you have an outdoor space, consider making a mini pond to attract thirsty creatures; for example, a large, clean plant pot filled with water. Just make sure there's a way for animals to get out if they fall in! Grass snakes are the biggest and most prolific snakes in the UK and are sometimes seen in ponds and canals where they feed on amphibians and fish.

At the seaside, the water is warm and seaweed is still plentiful. Jellyfish are a spectacular sight in July and August, especially the harmless 'moon' jellyfish, which can be seen in harbours and even in lochs – distinctive thanks to their translucent bell shape. Sadly, the spectacle of groups of jellyfish swarming together is becoming rarer thanks to rising sea temperatures. On the west coast of the UK, you might spot basking sharks – these huge, harmless sharks can grow up to eight metres long. They look like they could eat you whole, but these gentle giants' gaping mouths only collect plankton. In recent years, whale watching has taken off; minke whales are the most commonly seen species, spotted around the north of the UK and Ireland. Grey seals can be seen feeding close to the shore at the coast as well. And you can see dolphin pods around the UK, especially on the northeast coast of Scotland and southwest coast of England.

Thanks to conservation efforts, ospreys are thriving in the UK. In July, osprey chicks leave the nest, so this is a good time to try and spot them. Young peregrine falcons practise flying close to home before they, too, leave for good. Robins moult their feathers and keep a low profile in Summer but reappear in August with a new red coat – a sure sign we are in the latter half of the year. Barn owl sightings also peak in Summer; you might see them at dawn or dusk, stealthily hunting for food to feed their broods, sometimes producing two per Summer. At dusk, swifts can be spotted, ducking and diving around the rooftops, making their voices heard. Swallows and house martins gather more regularly as Summer wanes and their long journey nears: a certain sign that Autumn is on its way sooner rather than later.

BLACKBERRY PICKING

Nothing reminds us more of the march of time than the seasons, but the mindful activity of seasonal blackberry picking is, for me, a way to stop the clock and engage all the senses.

Blackberries are not, technically, a berry but an 'aggregate fruit' composed of small drupelets or stone fruit. They flower in late Spring and early Summer and can be found in the wild throughout Europe. They are incredibly vigorous and tolerate poor soils, meaning they rapidly colonise wasteland, ditches, scrubland, hedgerows and woods. Blackberries are considered a weed, yet they are an important part of ecosystems.

Picking blackberries is a popular pastime in many countries. They are well-liked thanks to their abundance and distinctive flavour. Have you ever stopped to notice how the blackberries ripen at different times? What about the subtle differences in their appearance and texture? Big, small, plump, some with lots of seeds and others with big, bloated bobbles. They all taste different too! Over time you will get to know the spots best for blackberries to snack on, for those suited to warming gently in a crumble and for the ones that are best saved for jam.

Humans have eaten blackberries for thousands of years. They have a long history of being preserved for wintertime and beyond in jellies, jams, wines and cordials. All parts of the plants, including the roots, leaves and bark, and particularly the tannin-rich leaves with their antibacterial properties, have also been used for centuries for medicinal purposes in Western cultures. The fruit and leaves have also been used to dye fabrics, and you can even make rope from the stems.

First appearing in August, blackberries herald the start of Autumn's fruits and can be picked until the beginning of October. According to British and Irish folklore, blackberries should not be picked after 'Devil Spits Day' – 10 or 11 October, depending on who you ask. This coincides with Old Michaelmas Day, the celebration of harvest's end. According to legend, on this day the devil fell from the skies into a blackberry bush (ouch) and cursed, scorched, stamped and spat on the fruits, rendering them inedible. Superstitious or not, the best berries can certainly be found before the first week of October, when wetter, cooler weather renders them inedible.

The simple, nostalgic pleasure of blackberrying is part of many children's stories such as the Brambly Hedge series. Otherwise in culture, the blackberry has a conflicting image. Brambles are often associated with dark things, traditionally regarded as the aforementioned devil's fruit.

FORAGING TIPS

Make sure you're prepared for picking: you will need dedication, gardening gloves, maybe even a small step ladder (or a tall friend) and a large plastic container to collect them in. My theory is that blackberries are so delicious because the ripest and juiciest are hardest won.

Forage safely and sustainably: look out for blackberry flowers in Summer to plan your foraging route ahead of time. Always pick fruit from above waist (and dog wee) height, and don't pick near busy roads or railways. For the best flavour, pick berries at the end of a sunny, warm afternoon.

When picking, the ripe, dark berries will be tastiest, but avoid over-ripe berries that immediately squash once picked, as they will make the rest of your haul go off more quickly. A few red or green berries are acceptable if you're making jam, as they are higher in pectin. Be sure to leave enough fruit for other foragers and the wildlife – vital for spreading seeds and continuing the cycle of life.

When you get home, process your haul as soon as possible to get the most of that fruity freshness before the berries start fermenting. Start by spreading the blackberries on a large tray to let any wildlife escape, then rinse them in a colander and use as desired.

There are so many different ways to use blackberries, from crumbles to pies, jams to jellies; raw or stewed, pickled or poached. The following recipes work with a variety of Autumn fruits and foraging finds – just adapt the levels of sugar to your taste, experiment and have fun!

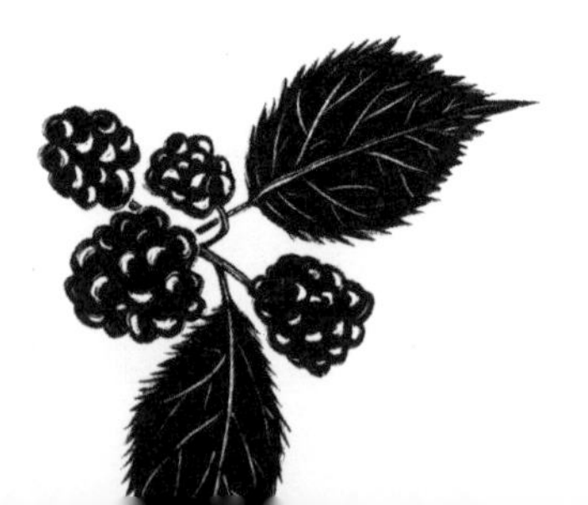

BLACKBERRY SHRUB

Shrubs or drinking vinegars are a retro way of preserving blackberries' intense flavour in pickled form. If you have a taste for sour things, then you will love this fruit-infused, non-alcoholic beverage. It can be made with all manner of seasonal fruits. The amount you make will depend on how much fruit you can forage.

YOU WILL NEED (1:1:1 RATIO)

Foraged fruit
Cider vinegar
Caster sugar

Set the oven to 110°C/Fan 100°C/Gas Mark ¼.

In a medium bowl, lightly mash the fruit to get the juices running.

Wash a glass jar or wide-necked bottle in warm water, then dry it in the oven for 20 minutes to sterilise. Allow to cool a little, then add the fruit.

In a pan over a medium–high heat, warm the vinegar until just boiling, then pour this over the fruit, leaving a little room at the top of the jar.

Cover, then set aside the fruit-filled vinegar and store it in a cool, dark place for anything from 24 hours to a few weeks to infuse.

When ready to use, strain out the fruit using a fine sieve (use the chilled fruit for salads or sauces). Pour the blackberry vinegar into a clean pan, then add the sugar.

Place over a low–medium heat and bring the vinegar-sugar mixture to the boil. Simmer until the sugar has dissolved.

Pour the shrub into a clean, sterilised jar or bottle and store it in the fridge. Serve diluted with soda water or use it in cocktails.

Note

The shrub will last for a good few months – but discard it if you see any signs of mould or if it starts to smell yucky.

BLACKBERRY FRUIT LEATHER

Making fruit 'leather' by drying fruit purées made with berries and orchard fruits dehydrates the fruit, intensifies its flavour and makes it last longer. Blackberries lend themselves to this recipe as their flavour is so distinctive – a delicious early Autumn snack for kids and grown-ups alike. If you want to eke out your haul, add the same quantity of cooking apples to blackberries.

YOU WILL NEED

Foraged blackberries, gently washed
Lemon juice, to taste
Spices (such as cinnamon or cardamom), to taste
Caster sugar (1⁄5 volume of fruit), or more to taste

Pre-heat the oven to its lowest temperature and line a large baking tray with greaseproof paper.

Note the weight of the blackberries (you will need it later), then place them in a large pan, covering with a little water. Warm over a low heat for 15–20 minutes, until the blackberries become soft and yielding.

Taste the blackberries and add a squeeze of lemon juice and a sprinkling of your desired spices, and the sugar (I find that around a fifth of the total weight of fruit generally works – it should still be a little tart). Taste and add more sugar and spice if needed.

Stir until the sugar has dissolved and the mixture has thickened enough to leave a clear patch on the bottom of the pan when you move the spoon through the mixture.

Strain into a large bowl and taste again, adding more sugar or spice, if needed.

Pour the mixture over the lined tray, thinly spreading it out to no more than 2–3mm thick.

Place the baking tray in a low oven until the purée has dried out: the timing depends on your oven temperature and how watery the blackberries were, but generally this can take up to 8 hours. (My oven goes as low as 35°C and took 12 hours, but at 110°C/Fan 100°C/Gas Mark 1⁄4 it took around 2 hours.)

When it is ready, the fruit will have completely dried out with no sticky patches left, will have a leathery texture and be easy to peel from the tray.

Once it has dried out, peel the fruit leather from the tray, cut it into strips and roll them up for storage in an airtight container in the fridge or freezer. The fruit leather will store in the fridge for around a month or in the freezer for a few months.

BLACKBERRY, CHOCOLATE & CARDAMOM CAKE

Chocolate and blackberries pair perfectly together, balancing rich and sharp flavours. I add cardamom into the mix to give the cake an aromatic, early Autumn twist, but if you're not keen, then you can just leave it out. This cake is delicious served cold with a pot of coffee or eaten warm with some double cream for an indulgent pudding. Granda didn't get to taste this one, but I know he would have loved it.

SERVES 6–8

- 120g unsalted butter, plus extra for greasing
- 120g caster sugar
- 2 tsp ground cardamom
- 2 large free-range eggs
- 100g self-raising flour
- 20g cocoa powder
- ½ tsp baking powder
- 2 tbsp milk
- 100g blackberries, halved if large
- 50g chocolate, chopped into small chunks
- 1 tbsp demerara sugar

Pre-heat the oven to 180°C/Fan 160°C/Gas Mark 4 and grease and line a 20cm cake tin.

In a bowl, cream the butter and sugar together until light and fluffy – about 5 minutes. Add the ground cardamom and beat again.

Add the eggs, one at a time, with a little flour.

Lightly fold in the rest of the flour and the cocoa powder and baking powder, then loosen with the milk.

Fold in half of the blackberries and half of the chocolate, then pour the mixture into the tin. Level the surface, then decorate the top with the rest of the blackberries and chocolate, lightly pressing them into the mixture.

Sprinkle the top of the mixture with the demerara sugar and carefully slide the cake tin into the oven, baking the cake for 40–45 minutes, until a skewer inserted in the middle comes out clean.

Leave the cake to cool for a few minutes in the tin, then remove it from the oven and allow it to cool completely on a wire rack.

MA

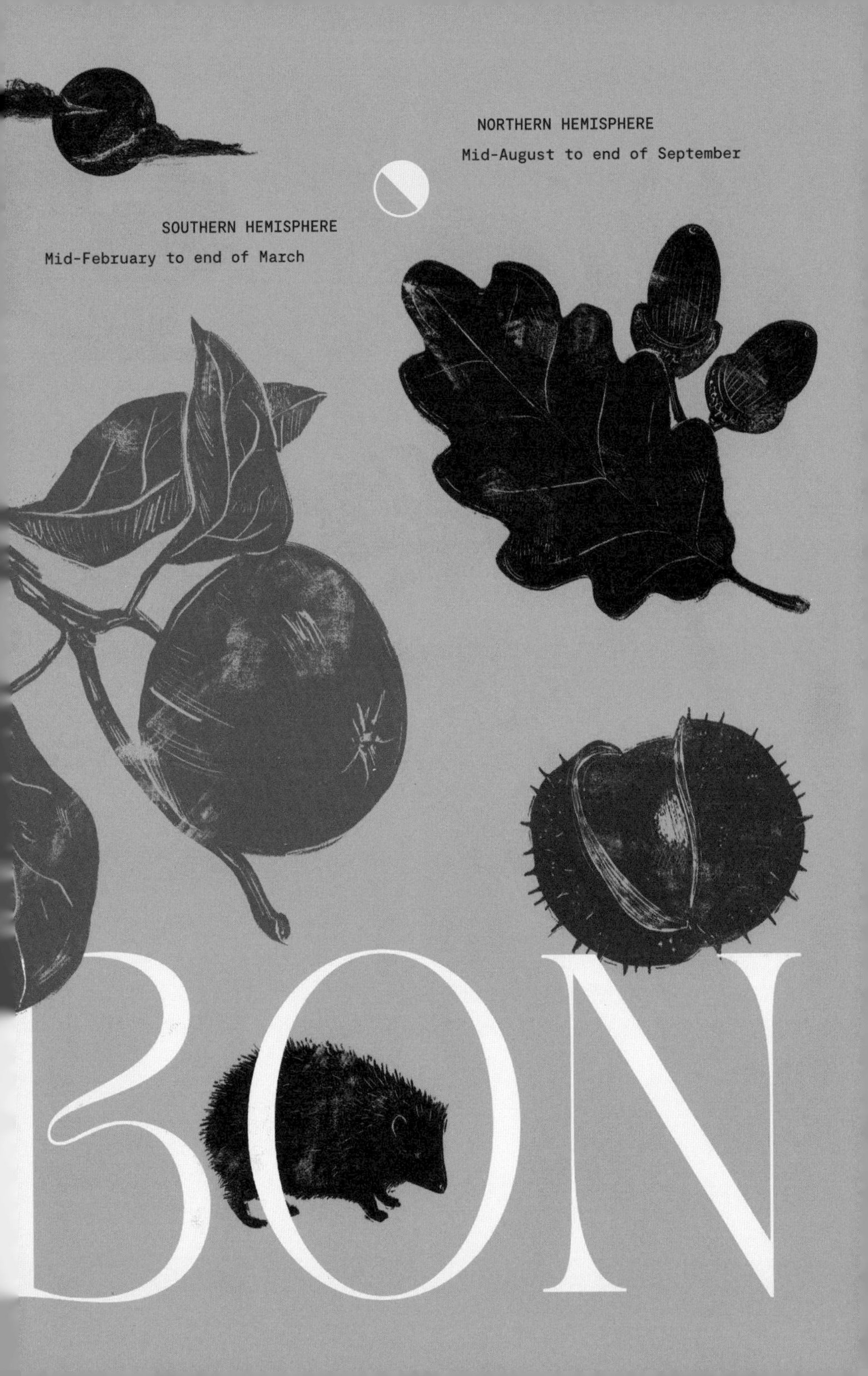
NORTHERN HEMISPHERE
Mid-August to end of September
SOUTHERN HEMISPHERE
Mid-February to end of March
BON

GIVING THANKS

The Celtic Wheel of the Year embraces balance in all things: light and dark, beginnings and endings, shaping the farming year around a comforting cycle. The festival of Mabon falls between 20 and 24 September, corresponding with the Autumn Equinox when day and night are of equal length once more. Versions of the festival have been celebrated for thousands of years, Mabon being the modern Pagan name for an ancient time that stood for balance. This second of the three harvest festivals, between Lùnastal and Samhain, is opposite Ostara at the Spring Equinox; it is sometimes known as the fruit harvest and is symbolised by the apple, representing beauty, youth and longevity. Mabon is a time of thanksgiving for the earth's harvest, which Celts traditionally shared with their deities in exchange for their blessings over the Winter months.

This is one of my favourite times in the Wheel of the Year. Golden sunshine and cold, crisp mornings; sandals and cardigans; the last barbecues and blankets. A long, languid farewell to warm, light, golden evenings, and a chance to savour a few final slow, sunny adventures. I might be biased as my birthday is in September, but beauty can be found in these contradictions. One year, Granda cut down my favourite tree, a tree of heaven, in the garden, as it was failing to thrive. Its leaves would turn the most spectacular highlighter hues in Autumn and at the time I was heartbroken to miss its transformation. However, it was a lesson in acceptance, Mabon being a time of change and letting things go.

> AND CHANGE IS CERTAINLY IN THE AIR: ALL AROUND THE FAINTEST FLICKER OF RUSSET AND AMBER APPEAR FROM LEAVES ON THE CUSP OF A SPECTACULAR TRANSFORMATION.

The first tree to feel a shiver is the horse chestnut, then the beech, maple and silver birch. Conkers are abundant and elderberries are ripening, heavy with purple-black fruit. The hedgerow begins to fill with the first hawthorns, with rosehips and plentiful blackberries.

The breeze has a freshness and the first whiffs of wood burners on colder days. We find ourselves reaching for a light coat, or maybe a scarf. There's a continuing new-term feeling, the memory of new stationery, crisp ironed shirts, shiny shoes and too-big blazers deeply ingrained in our collective consciousness. To me, this time from Lùnastal to Mabon feels more like a new year than January, signalling fresh starts and organising for the season ahead.

It's tempting to throw yourself headfirst into the anticipation of all the autumnal goodness to come, powered by that fresh, new season energy – but so much beauty can be found in these in between moments of quiet magic.

Seasonal Celebrations at Home

I find the turn of each season a good time to check in with myself and those around me. These days I feel the seasonal shift in my bones – I become restless, simultaneously brimming with ideas and feeling tired and lethargic as my circadian rhythms adapt to the shortening days and return towards darkness. Pay attention to what your body tells you; get into good sleep routines with earlier nights and healthier habits that might have gone awry during the Summer months. Set aside time for that new project (a shiny new notebook or pen always helps) and reflect on where you are now and where you want to be next season. Note down some small, manageable steps that will take you closer to your goal and, above all, be kind to yourself.

Saying Goodbye to Summer

Long, lazy Summer days are coming to an end. Enjoy a few last hurrahs, weather-permitting, and eat outside whenever possible: have picnics, head to the beach, tick off the last items on your Summer bucket list. Make a mindful ritual of sorting your Summer memories: whether that's collected objects, photographs or other visuals or souvenirs. Put that local crockery from your holiday in pride of place in the kitchen, print photographs and display them in simple clip frames. Like a physical gratitude journal, these sunny mementos will be comforting reminders on grey, endless Winter days that Summer will come again.

As well as time to reflect, at the beginning of each season I like to get organised for the months ahead. First, set aside time to declutter and sort the Summer detritus that has accumulated over the months you were busier or away from home. Sort through your Summer clothes (did you love that bikini/top/skirt this Summer? If not, chances are you won't next Summer, so donate them to charity). Organise paperwork; take stock of what's in the larder; tidy cluttered surfaces and shelves. Then welcome in the new season: air blankets and throws; wash your knitwear, slowly restock the larder and invest in some beeswax or soy candles for the colder months ahead – or even make your own (see page 22).

Early Autumn Foraging

This is a golden time for foraging with so much wild food ripe for the picking. Remember to forage responsibly: ask the landowner's permission, take sparingly from different areas (certainly no more than a third of whatever you forage), and leave plenty for the wildlife. Spend the afternoon in the kitchen with your finds tending simmering pots and pans – your house will smell like Autumn in an instant. Elderberries are filled with vitamins A and C and studies show they're more effective at beating flu than over-the-counter drugs. Elderberry tonic is good for you, too, and delicious. I was first introduced to the tipple by my friend and foraging expert Alison Henderson on a sunny September day in the wilds of East Lothian, and now I make my own elderberry cordial every Mabon. Spend time stripping the berries from the stems with a fork or your fingers (this part is very therapeutic), cover with water and simmer until the berries yield, mashing them to encourage all the juice from within. Strain through a muslin and measure your juice. Pour it into a fresh pan with 200g of sugar to every 300ml juice and the juice of half a citrus fruit (I like orange). At this stage you could add Autumn spices for a seasonal kick – I love the aroma of a few cardamom pods. Simmer until the sugar has dissolved then boil until the mixture has reduced to a syrupy consistency, around 20 minutes (though this depends on how much juice you extracted). Strain into a sterilised bottle and serve diluted with hot water for a warming autumnal drink or drizzle, neat, on top of porridge. It will keep for a few months in the fridge or you can freeze portions in an ice cube tray to keep it for longer.

Early Autumn Evening Strolls

Enjoy the early Autumn light that cloaks everything in a golden glow shortly before sunrise and sunset. Notice how the light reveals the unexpected, or how it casts your usual walk with a magic haze and draws attention to things usually unnoticed. Capture the seasonal transition by going on a photo walk or take your sketchbook with you. Or why not collect some nature finds and photograph or sketch them when you get home? You could even combine the three like a modern version of Edith Holden's *The Country Diary of an Edwardian Lady* – sketches, journal jottings and seasonal quotes.

Harvest Festival

Since Pagan times, thanks have been given for successful harvests, with the harvest festival traditionally held on the Sunday closest to the Harvest Moon (which is the full moon closest to the Autumn Equinox) in late September or early October. Traditional harvest loaves and corn dollies are made, and the table is decorated with baskets of Autumn fruit for communal feasts and merriment. This is a time of giving, too: donate to a local charity or a food bank to help those in need. Contact food banks near you to find out what is needed locally; they can identify people in crisis and provide emergency food to support those living in poverty.

Celebrate the Autumn Equinox

Although meteorological Autumn is technically on 1 September in the Northern Hemisphere, the Autumn Equinox, Mabon, or astronomical Autumn feels a lot more like the beginning of Autumn to me. It's a great excuse to decorate the house with pretty, seasonal gatherings – conkers, changing leaves, acorns and dried hydrangea heads. This is a day of balance: take time to nurture those things that bring harmony to your life. Hosting a themed dinner party is a great way to welcome in the new season; get everyone to bring a pot of something seasonal (organised beforehand to ensure a range of goodies) and share together – outside if you can.

AUTUMN WREATH

Decorating for your harvest celebration is a fun way to see in the new season. A wreath isn't just for Christmas: a simple, woven wreath base is a perfectly versatile addition to your home that can be decorated and updated for every season. It doesn't have to go on your door either: hung over a mantel or on a hook, wreaths are a simple and effective way to add natural texture and interest to the home.

I live in a tenement flat with a communal stair so I hang my wreath inside – either on my peg rail that I thrifted at a vintage fair for a tenner, that now hangs on the only bare wall in my flat, on the back of a door on a vintage hook, or perched precariously on a pin above my mantel in the kitchen. I have a few wreath bases on rotation now, some that I have made (like the one on page 134) and a couple of cheat's pre-made ones, crafted from willow, that are easy to store flat in a drawer and bring out to decorate when I fancy a quick craft. I find it nigh on impossible not to gather branches, bracken or other nature finds on walks. I also find myself, sometimes inadvertently, drying out flowers and foliage. I become overly attached to these bits of nature, storing them in vases on top of my kitchen dresser, which my partner calls my 'lovely dead crap'. Please don't tell me I'm the only one who does this?!

Something about the shape of a branch or perfect dried skeleton of a Summer flower or fragility of a seed head has my heart, even more so than their fresh counterparts. Do beware decorating or hanging your seasonal wreath next to unattended candles, however. I am a notoriously clumsy crafter and have been known to accidentally set my projects alight when taking photos. The worst has got to be the scent of burning heather, though the charring did create an interesting finish! On a serious note, dried flowers and foliage do set alight easily so make sure that the candles are well out of reach.

Making your own wreath is easier than you might think, and there's something so therapeutic about the repetitive motion of weaving twigs together. It's a great excuse to go out foraging, too, and a lovely way to display your finds.

FORAGING FOR MATERIALS: HINTS AND TIPS

For the wreath base, look for fallen young twigs that you can easily shape. Ignore anything that has been dead for a while – it will be too brittle and snap as soon as you look at it, never mind try to bend it. A good time to source these twigs is after a storm or, if you have a garden, when pruning your trees in Spring or Summer – you could stock up and make your bases then. The stems of willow, dogwood or climbers are flexible and easier to work with too.

The length of your largest twig will dictate the size of your wreath, when bent into a full circle. If the rest are shorter it won't matter, as you will weave them round the initial base – I find a variety of lengths creates a pleasing texture.

You can decorate your base with whatever you can find – just remember anything fragile, like leaves, will dry out and curl up quite quickly. However, this is still pretty!

Tougher berries like those of the rowan will last for a few days before going a little wrinkly, though again this can add interesting texture. If you want to preserve the ripe berries, you can find glycerine in most chemists or big supermarket bakery aisles and make a 1:2 solution of glycerine: water. Keep the berries or leaves submerged in the solution for a few days to preserve them, then dry before use.

I usually aim to collect foraging finds that will dry out beautifully and make my wreath everlasting. Honesty (*Lunaria*) seed heads, pine cones and heather flowers dry well naturally without intervention. Avoid anything with a soft stem or delicate flowers that even once preserved may be too fragile to withstand the wreath-making process.

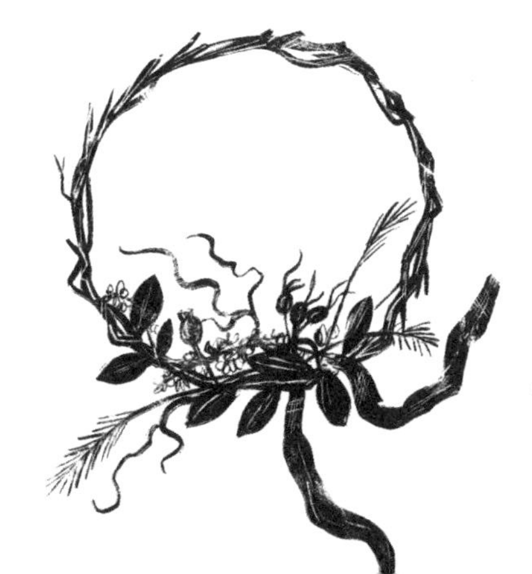

AUTUMN WREATH BASE

This everlasting wreath base can be decorated and re-decorated over and over again. Once it has been made and dried out it becomes inflexible, so may be a little trickier to adapt but it will keep its shape well. The number of twigs you need will depend on the desired size and thickness of your wreath. For a 30cm diameter ring, ensure your largest twig is about 1m long.

YOU WILL NEED

Long, bendy twigs
Secateurs or scissors
Approx. 2m florist's wire (it comes in rolls but will last for years; ask your local florist)
Foraging finds, to decorate
Ribbon (see notes)
Hook or peg rail, for hanging (see notes)

Form the base by curving the largest twig into a circle. Ensure the ends overlap a little and firmly secure in place with florist's wire. Don't worry if your base is a little wonky – you will shape it into a better circle as you add layers.

Loosely weave a second twig around the frame, securing with more wire at the start and end.

Add more twigs, following a loose spiral around the base and securing with wire as necessary, all the while lightly bending the wreath into a more circular shape.

Keep adding twigs: after a while you can simply tuck them in, which will hide the wire you've used. Include a few stems going in the other direction to add fullness and to prevent the wreath from being too uniform.

Step back and assess where you want to put the foraging finds. (This is an opportunity to cover up any less-than-perfect areas!)

Now decorate your wreath, starting with bulkier items such as pine cones towards the back (so they do not crush anything more delicate). To create volume, add flora in little bundles tied together with florist's wire, and secure to the base.

Feed more delicate stems through the twigs of the wreath to hide the wire: gently pull them through until they catch at the back of the wreath and weave the stems into the base to secure.

Gradually build your decoration, stepping back occasionally to monitor the balance of the wreath. I find it looks more impactful to cover one half of the wreath (top or bottom) rather than the whole thing.

Step back and admire your handiwork! Hang by securing a coloured ribbon around the top of the wreath, tied in a bow.

Hang up the wreath to dry out; the timing of this depends on the type of foliage you have used, but it generally takes a few days to a week. When you want to reuse the base (which will have become hard and light) strip your wreath outside (keep the wire to use again) so you don't make a mess of dead pine needles all over your kitchen – like I did!

Notes

I source naturally dyed ribbons from Kent-based business The Natural Dyeworks. Ros hand dyes each of the ribbons from locally foraged, natural ingredients and creates a mind-boggling array of beautiful colours inspired by nature.

I am always on the lookout for old hooks that can be picked up for a few pounds from vintage fairs and attached to the back of a door. A peg rail is beautiful as well as useful; you can even buy pegs online and a piece of pre-cut wood and make your own. And if you're renting, you can buy transparent, self-adhesive hooks that can be easily removed when you move out – just make sure you get the right size for the weight you plan to hang and that you follow the instructions to hang it properly (I learnt this to my cost).

APPLE & STAR ANISE CAKE

Apples are traditionally seen as symbol of Mabon. I like to make a cake with the first, crisp new season apples for harvest celebrations – their flavour is like nothing else. Gran used to make a delicious apple cake with chunks of fresh fruit. This is my nod to the family tradition with a subtly spicy twist, delicious served warm with custard.

SERVES APPROX. 8

- 100g butter
- ½ tsp ground star anise (buy pre-ground or grind your own in a spice grinder)
- 75g caster sugar
- 25g dark brown sugar
- 2 large free-range eggs
- 75g self-raising flour
- 25g spelt flour
- 2 apples, one chopped into chunks and one thinly sliced (skin on)
- 1 tbsp demerara sugar

Pre-heat the oven to 180°C/Fan 160°C/Gas Mark 4 and grease and line a 20cm cake tin.

In a bowl, cream the butter, spice and sugars together with a wooden spoon until light and fluffy.

Beat in the eggs, one at a time, with a little of the self-raising flour between each addition.

Gently fold in the remaining self-raising flour and the spelt flour, followed by the chopped apple.

Pour the mixture into the prepared cake tin. Decorate the top with the thinly sliced apple, gently pressing it into the surface.

Sprinkle with the demerara and bake for 45 minutes until a skewer inserted in the middle comes out clean.

Remove from the oven and leave to cool on a wire rack.

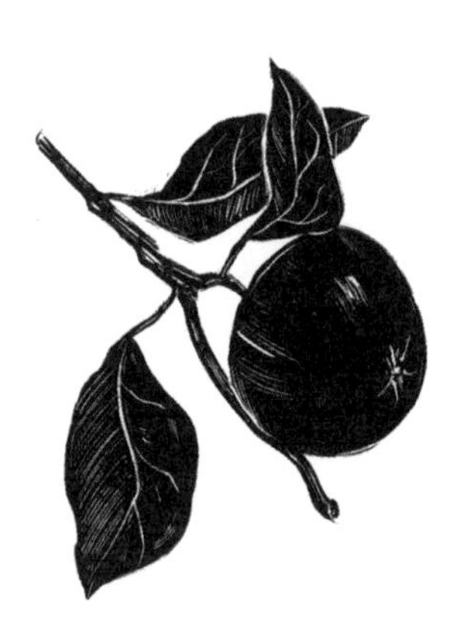

Seasonal Celebrations of Nature

Mabon is a magical transitional time: often, a heady combination of sunshine and late Summer rain encourages abundance. One of my fondest childhood memories is of the nature table at school where we were invited to show and tell our Autumn finds. I hunted high and low for conkers, to no avail. Eventually Gran surprised me with a box of the elusive conkers, nestled inside, that she had foraged for me on a walk. I brought them to the nature table with pride.

Recently I worked out where to find conkers and I now host my own nature table at school: I challenge my pupils to find the biggest, shiniest or smallest, cutest conkers to display in my classroom. The innocent glee the competition inspires always restores my faith in humanity.

The trees, of course, show the main sign that Autumn is on its way. The canopy and leaves on any exposed branches change colour first. Nuts and berries are plentiful on trees and in hedgerows as they begin to shed their fruits. Rosehips and hawthorns are ripening in the upper branches and the first sloes might begin to appear.

Early green acorns can already be found under oak trees, while the rest ripen on the tree and turn brown. Gradually, then suddenly all at once, conkers fall from the horse chestnut tree. Have a traditional conker competition (safety goggles optional) or simply see who can find the biggest and shiniest seasonal treasures. Mushrooms make an appearance in grassy areas, particularly after early Autumn rains. See which fungi you can find in your local mixed woodland; you might be surprised. Make sure you take a guide to help you identify them and never eat anything that you're unsure of.

Warm days coax out butterflies and insects such as common darters, while late flowering ivy provides food for hoverflies, red admiral butterflies and late bumblebees such as the ivy bee (*Colletes hederae*) with its very stripy abdomen. When the sun is out, see if you can spot them buzzing around the ivy. Plenty of Autumn moths can be seen on the changing leaves, echoing the season's colour palette in brilliant yellows and even pinks; they are so well camouflaged you might find them hard to spot! Hedgehogs begin to think of hibernation and squirrels start collecting nuts to store for Winter.

Migration is a common theme, with some visitors leaving as others arrive. Geese, ducks and wading birds overwinter in the UK, arriving from the north and east, as do tiny goldcrests, flycatchers and redstarts. You are likely to hear the sound of geese before you see them moving in their elegant V-shaped formations. Yellow-browed warblers migrate from the forests of Siberia and are increasingly common in the UK thanks to changing migratory routes. Birds seeking warmer climes leave our shores to head south for Winter, gathering in groups before they depart; look out for them on electric wires over roads. Take time to observe the collective excitement of swallows, house martins and sand martins, and the conversational calls between family groups. The swifts are first to depart, while swallows and martins leave close to the Autumn Equinox.

The Harvest Moon is a special full moon closest to the Equinox. The low angle of the moon's orbit in relation to the Earth's horizon creates significantly earlier moonrises – a phenomenon called the Harvest Moon Effect. Traditionally this meant farmers could harvest crops for longer in the evenings. The Equinox is also a prime time for those in the Northern Hemisphere to see the aurora borealis (Northern Lights) at high latitudes, thanks to greater geomagnetic activities at these times of balance in Spring and Autumn.

Sea water is at its warmest, heated by the Summer sun. This prompts rapid growth of seaweeds, at its height, and marine organisms are busy – look in rock pools for crabs, shrimp, limpets and more. So much diversity in such a tiny ecosystem. In some rivers, salmon begin to travel upstream to breed while in lakes and reservoirs you might spot ducks such as drake mallards moulting, shedding their emerald green Summer feathers, used to attract a mate, for drab brown ones to avoid attracting predators over Winter.

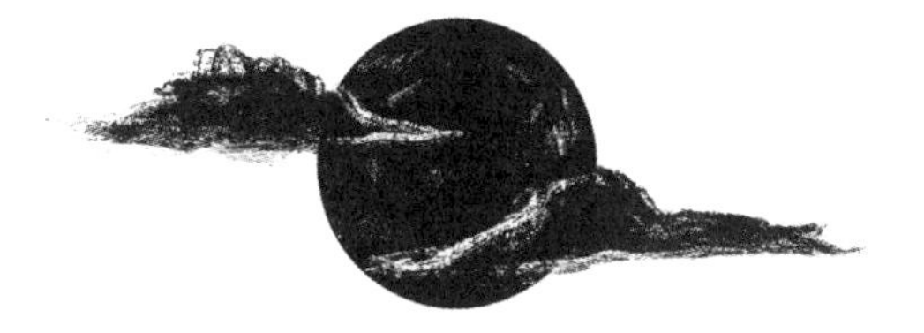

FOREST BATHING

We all know nature is good for us, but in the hustle and bustle of day-to-day life we can forget the restorative power of a simple walk in the woods. Something about the scale of a forest grounds us and reminds us of our place in the universe. A study by Heriot-Watt University and the University of Edinburgh found that walking in a green space for just twenty-five minutes triggers a meditative state and enhances mood. Forest bathing is a way to focus on the here and now, to engage all the senses in the process of noticing. What colours can you see? What can you smell? Inhale the sweet, fresh air, the scent of pine needles and distant streams. Feel the mossy ground beneath your feet and gaze up into the colourful, changing canopy. Observe the small details of nature around you. Breathe.

With younger classes, I like to play a game of making a 'sensory poem', and sound is our way into this task. I ask the class to stand beneath the trees and shut their eyes. I ask, 'What can you hear? Open your eyes and write down the words that pop into your head.' You might be surprised at how poetic the results are. Classes never look at trees in quite the same way again.

Forest History and Folklore

There's a reason why the woods have their own quiet magic, especially around Mabon. Many individual forests are associated with specific myths and legends as well as art and literature, from Robin Hood and Sherwood Forest to Birnam Wood and Macbeth.

And it's no wonder when many of our individual trees are associated with different magical stories and often linked to life and death. The ash tree was thought to have healing properties: newborns were fed ash sap and the mountain ash or rowan tree was thought to house fairies. The ancient Celts associated the hazelnut tree with wisdom and aspen wood with protection. Birch species are connected with fertility and purification as they are often the first trees to come into leaf in the springtime and among the last to lose their leaves. Elm is associated with the afterlife in both Celtic and Greek mythology and the yew tree is seen as a symbol of death and resurrection in Celtic culture – the reason you will often find this ancient tree in and around graveyards.

So, with their individual magic, it is unsurprising that forests themselves are seen as spiritual places, home to fairies and sprites, demons and devils: a subtle space between this world and the next. There's certainly something otherworldly about them, and all the more so around Mabon.

About Forest Bathing

In recent years, the Japanese practice of 'shinrin-yoku' (taking in the forest atmosphere) has grown in popularity as a form of meditation. The term emerged in the 1980s as a way to escape the sped-up pace of modern life and the growing role of technology, as well as to reconnect with nature. With their peaceful atmosphere and symbolic physical link back through the centuries, it's no wonder that forests and woodlands have a prominent role in many cultures' grounding practices, including for the Celts.

During each of the festivals of the Wheel of the Year, the Celts took to nature to celebrate. The changing energies reflected in the natural world are felt nowhere more keenly than the forest. The ancient practice of forest bathing is a sensory form of meditation: taking a moment of quiet in the trees to bring calm through observing nature and deep breathing. My friend Diana is a qualified forest bathing instructor. She explains it as 'using techniques to slow down, enhance the senses and build your connection'. This is more than just a walk in the woods: it's about engaging with your surroundings and grounding yourself in the here and now.

Although I live in the middle of the city, I am lucky to live near my own woodland escape. It seems completely incongruous, but just off the main road in one of the main arteries out of Edinburgh is a country lane that leads into the back of the Hermitage of Braid and Blackford Hill Local Nature Reserve. Just minutes from the hustle and bustle of the city I can follow the path along the Braid Burn (a small stream) and wander under the elm, ash and sycamore, birch, rowan and beech trees.

TIPS

- Despite its name, forest bathing requires no swimming costume, goggles or swimming cap – in fact, the less 'stuff' you bring with you the better! Leave your phone at home or switch it off to remove the distraction and tempting chirp of notifications.
- Aim to visit at a quiet time when the woods are likely to be undisturbed and you can concentrate fully on the moment.
- Start by taking long, deep breaths. I find that inhaling for seven seconds then out for eleven makes me breathe more deeply into my abdomen.
- Slow down: this isn't a race. Move at a deliberately slow pace so that you can observe more around you.
- Stop periodically and either stand or sit to take in your surroundings using all five senses. Breathe in the scent of citrusy pine trees. Savour the freshness of the air. Focus, too, on how the forest makes you feel.
- Try to avoid thinking about what you've left behind, that unanswered email or pressing item on your to-do list. If your mind drifts, gently bring it back to the present by acknowledging that your brain is human and has wandered, and by observing your surroundings and engaging your senses once again. What can you see below your feet? What can you hear in the distance? You might just be surprised by what you notice.
- Studies show that the colours of nature are soothing – there's a reason that shades of green rarely go out of fashion in interiors. Notice the subtle differences in shape and colour of the leaves.
- Stay as long as you are able. Research recommends up to two hours for a completely immersive forest bathing experience, but even short bursts of such focused meditation will make a big difference to your wellbeing, and you can build up to longer bathing sessions over time.
- If you can't get to a forest, studies show that even observing images of forests or listening to their sounds can have a similar soothing effect. You can find lots online.
- Heck, just stare at a tree if you can do nothing else! I find great calm in observing the seasonally changing profile of the silver birch tree outside my window.

Forest Bathing Activities

As well as mindful meditation, a few other activities can help keep you focused on the natural surroundings. A nature trail is a fun task, with children or not: come up with a list of flora and fauna to spot on your woodland walk, or even collect some specimens (carefully and sustainably) for a nature table. A basket is a must to hold the precious cargo, and a homemade list ready for recording finds is just the ticket. I try to seek out a leaf in each colour – gold, amber and russet – conkers and hazelnuts, pine cones and helicopter seeds, beech nuts and acorns.

Refuelling on such jaunts is also essential – and it is the official start of hot chocolate season. It's well worth investing in a local chocolatier's hot chocolate blend if you can find one – or if you can't get your hands on any, you can make your own. Measure a mug-full of milk into a small pan and grate in a couple of tablespoons of good quality chocolate. If you like, you could add a chilli into the mix to infuse and add some warming spice and a dash of vanilla for sweetness. Heat until the mixture is just about to boil, stirring constantly until bubbles form on the surface. Make sure you watch it like a hawk as it can boil over instantly, and trust me, spilt milk is a pain to shift from your hob! Strain into your favourite flask (if using the chilli, otherwise just pour it straight in) and bring a couple of enamel mugs with you to enjoy, perched on a tree trunk, to warm cold hands.

AUTUMN LEAF CRAFT

The changing leaves are all the more precious for their fleeting beauty and resistance to preservation. Perhaps nature is trying to tell us something? However, Autumn leaves are such fun to craft with and these few tips can make them last a little longer.

First and foremost, the main joy is in collecting the most beautiful Autumn leaves you can find on your mindful nature walk. English Oak trees are not as common where I live, so I delight in finding their curved leaves with distinctive, symmetrical lobes and ripe acorns when I do come across them, more commonly in the Borders and Perthshire during day trips. I clean any dirt from the leaves, then dry and press them underneath heavy books for at least twenty-four hours.

They're ready to craft with as you please after that – I use washi tape to secure them to the window, arranging them in a pattern of different sizes, colours and shapes and securing them top and bottom to make a seasonal display. This lets the light through and illuminates their Autumn colours even more. Embrace their fleeting nature and the organic shapes they form as they dry out and begin to curl.

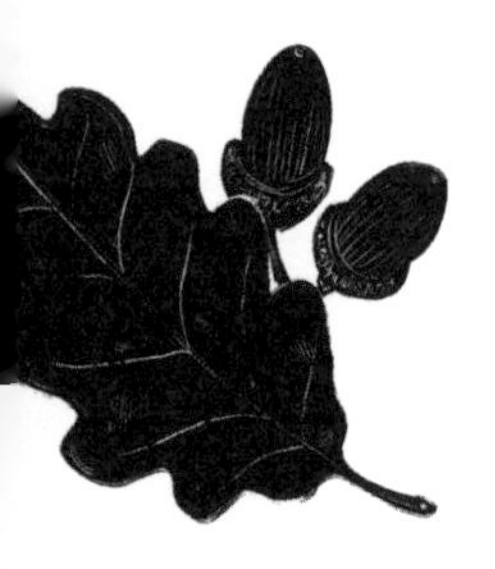

PAPER LEAF SWAG

I know that not everyone is lucky enough to live where there is a spectacular Autumn transformation, and that nature's palette can be more subdued. Sometimes, you have to make your own Autumn colour!

YOU WILL NEED

Large, flat brush
Red and yellow watercolour paints (cheap palettes are fine – you don't need fancy paint!)
Sheets of thick A4 paper (at least three – one for each colour – but use more depending on how many leaves you want to make and how big your reference leaf is)
2 jars of water
China plate, for mixing colours
Leaf
Pencil
Cardboard (you could recycle e.g. a cereal box)
Scissors
Hole punch
30cm-long branch
Twine

With the brush, paint wide, horizontal strokes at the top of the paper.

Clean your brush in the first jar of water, then dip it in the second clean jar of water and brush along your last stroke, overlapping slightly to dilute the colour.

Repeat as you work down the page, so the colour becomes less intense, until you reach the bottom of the paper.

Change your water, repeat with the other colour on a fresh piece of paper and leave to dry.

Mix red and yellow together on the plate to make orange. Change your water again. Repeat the colour wash with the orange paint on a third piece of paper, then leave to dry.

While everything is drying, draw round your leaf onto the cardboard. Cut around the leaf to make a template.

Turn your coloured paper over and draw round the template, trying to fit as many shapes on the page as possible.

Cut around the leaf shapes with your scissors, then set to one side.

If you want to make your leaves more lifelike, draw veins on the white side of the paper, pushing the pencil hard to make an indentation on the front.

Punch a hole on one end of each leaf (do this on the same end of each leaf).

Take a leaf and the branch and decide how far down you want the leaf to hang. Cut the twine to this length. Tie one end of the twine to the leaf end and the other to the branch. Repeat until you have hung all the leaves – a mixture of different lengths works well.

Attach a long piece of twine to each end of the branch and hang your swag against the wall or on a hook.

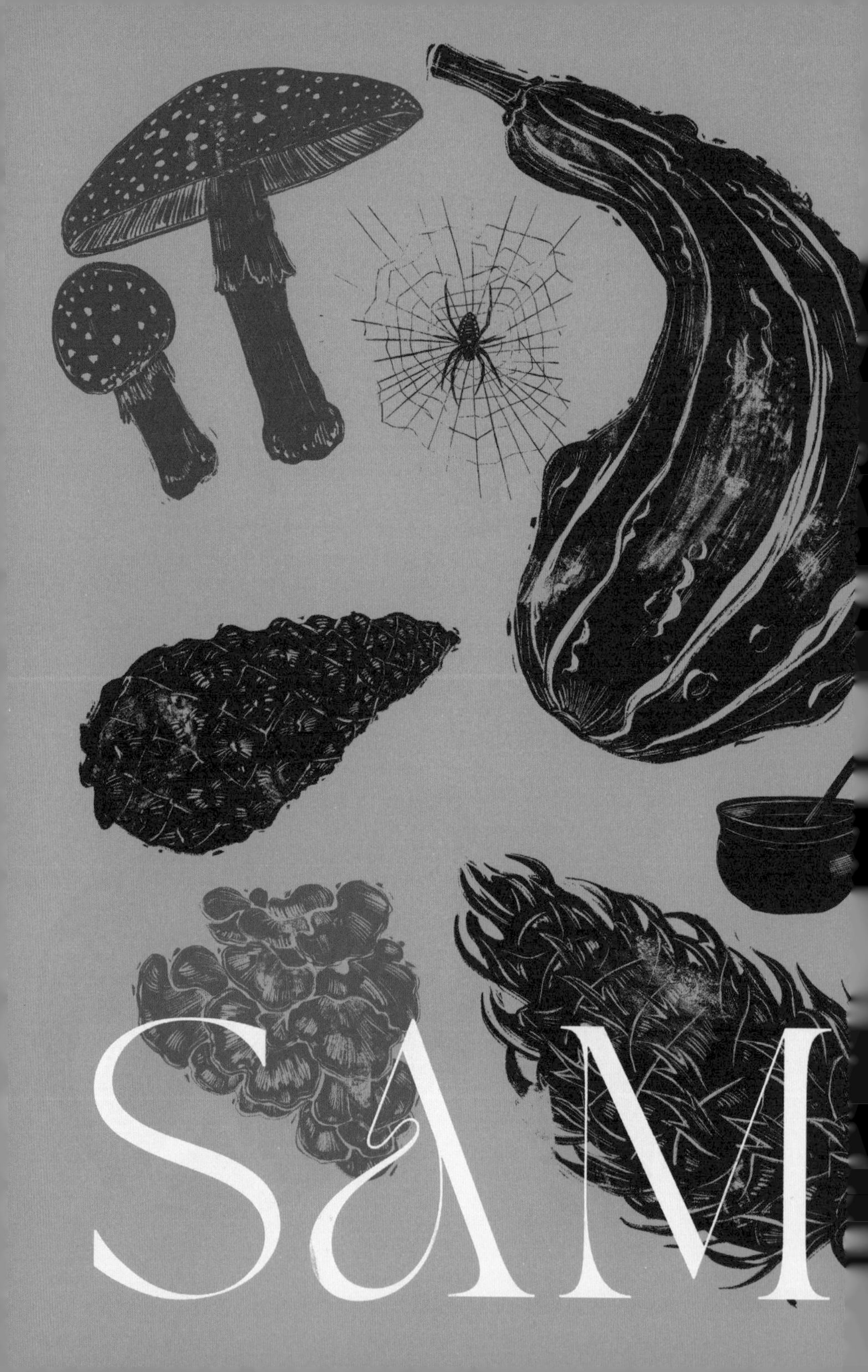
SAM

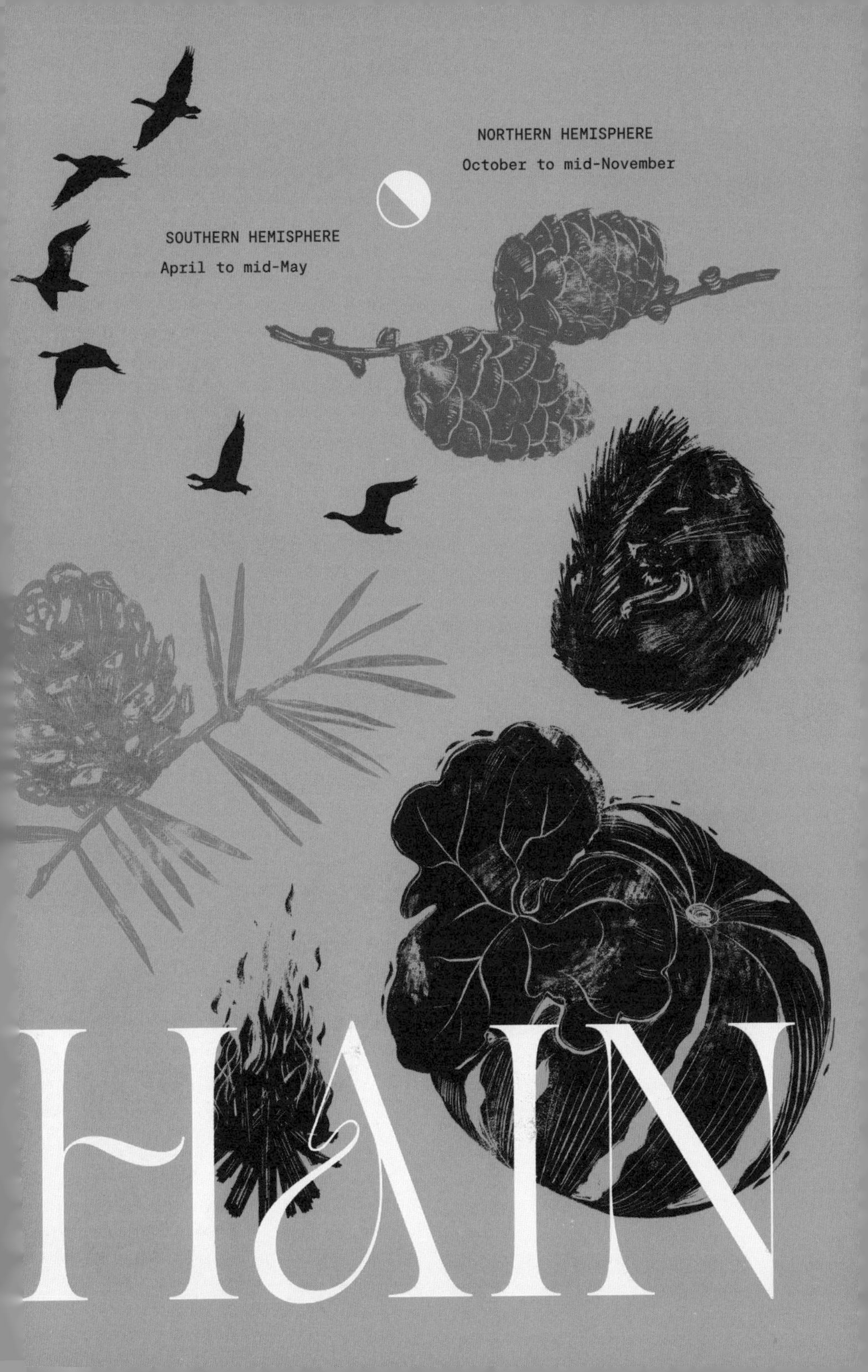
NORTHERN HEMISPHERE
October to mid-November
SOUTHERN HEMISPHERE
April to mid-May
HAIN

DARKNESS DESCENDS

Autumn weeks tick by, and the days are slowly creeping shorter. In the Celtic Wheel of the Year, Samhain (pronounced 'Sah-wane') is regarded as the 'Celtic Halloween'. While it tends to coincide with contemporary Halloween celebrations and, indeed, is the origin of many of them (as I will explore in this chapter) it is also the third and final harvest festival and the beginning of Winter in the Celtic calendar. Gradually at first, then suddenly all at once: as the Celtic Wheel turns, we find ourselves embraced by the darkness.

Too often darkness is associated with negativity, and certainly the limited daylight hours and lack of sunshine take their toll. However, I've found a subtle shift in mindset helped me to reclaim this time and savour the darkness. Embracing our inner child is key: transporting ourselves back to childhood and experiencing the awe of our first Autumns: the pure, unadulterated magic of transforming trees, first frosts, fairytale mushrooms, bare branches and berries.

> WHETHER YOU'RE IN THE COUNTRYSIDE OR THE CITY, SO MUCH DAILY MAGIC CAN BE FOUND – YOU JUST HAVE TO STOP, SLOW DOWN, AND LOOK AROUND.

This is easier said than done in our hectic lives, I know, but there's something about Autumn that invites us to do so, perhaps because of its fleeting beauty as our surroundings seem to change and evolve; or perhaps it's our inner clock, reacting to the waning light, that urges us to slow and take stock before we hunker down. I love my walk to work around Samhain: I always notice something new that grounds me in the moment, whether it's the first rowan tree leaves that have turned or the last hydrangea that has dried to the perfect dusky purple. The quiet wonder of nature. This is when I really start craving comfort: I finally switch on the heating – usually resisted until at least Samhain – for an hour or two and savour it all the more for the wait. Blankets become a feature in every room, and knitwear is a daily staple once again.

Memories of my childhood Samhain celebrations are some of the most vivid. Mum would always admirably commit to a decorative theme, with simple crêpe paper garlands and decorations drawn by my brother and me. We would save up the special candles and gather round the table as they burnt – their scent of cardamom, coriander and cinnamon transports me right back. We would eat simple yet special vegetable-centred suppers, and these inspire my own gatherings today, making the most of seasonal Scottish ingredients and warm hospitality.

Time in the kitchen soothes the soul: a bubbling pot of jam; squash roasting in the oven; tea warming on the stove. At this time of year, heartier foods call to us: a pan of soup, warming stew, hotpot, risottos, pasta bakes, pies and pastries – the list of comfort foods is endless. Seasonal spice tantalises tastebuds and, of course, the ubiquitous pumpkin features in all manner of makes and bakes.

The wind whistles down the chimney. A Samhain feast beckons.

I like to make evenings special, even if I'm on my own: as soon as I get home I light candles and turn on fairy lights; and after finishing my marking, I cook something comforting before curling up in a cosy corner with a book and homemade hot chocolate.

It may feel like the world is willing us to hurtle through the season headfirst into the festive countdown, but there is so much more to Autumn than just a few weeks. Making the most of the season you're in is key when darkness descends.

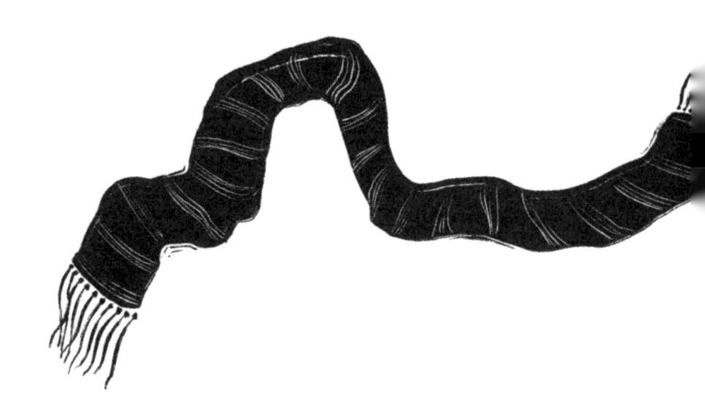

Seasonal Celebrations at Home

Celts from Scotland, Ireland and the Isle of Man celebrated Samhain from the evening of 31 October through to 1 November to mark the halfway point between the Autumn Equinox, Mabon, and the Winter Solstice, Yule. Great gatherings and feasts marked the supposedly fluid boundaries between the spirit and human worlds. Although many of these rituals were not recorded until the Modern Era, there are anecdotal reports of bonfire blessings, offerings and livestock slaughter (in a bid to appease the spirits). I've known other families to set a separate place at the table for the souls of dead relatives during Samhain, and some people think the tradition of guising (trick or treating) was a means of disguise against fairies.

Chasing Light

Celebrations of light and fire are ubiquitous at this time – the triumph of light over darkness, good over evil, is a motif across cultures. There's a reason so many late Autumn and Winter festivities, including Samhain, revolve around these themes, bringing cheer at this all-encompassing dark time. A bonfire – with or without fireworks – is a failsafe way to do just that, watching the flames as night descends, curled in blankets and talking over the crackling logs. The art of lighting a fire teaches patience, and lessons can be learnt from the fire itself: built too big, it will rapidly burn out; a long, slow burn provides the best warmth. Cooking on an open fire can take you back to basics; even toasting marshmallows or – a recent revelation – cooking apples in foil provides primitive pleasure. To make them, when the fire dies down, core your apples and stuff them with brown sugar, a knob of butter, and cinnamon; or, for a healthier option, dates soaked in boiling water then drained and mashed. You could also add dried fruit or chopped nuts. Wrap the apples individually in foil and cook them for around 10 minutes tucked beneath the embers. Be sure not to cook them for too long or they will explode! Handle with care and watch out for the steam on opening.

Squash Watch

Samhain coincides with squash season. Visiting a pumpkin patch is an American tradition that seems to have firmly made its way across the pond. Photo opportunities aside (no judgement here), it's well worth finding out if there's such a spot nearby. While supermarkets now stock different kinds of pumpkin, they are often grown for aesthetics rather than taste – not to mention that they're pricey. Local farmers are passionate about their fare and often have the best local, culinary pumpkin varieties, as well as the iconic orange giants, plus more and more are opening their fields and letting you pick your own. It's now an annual tradition in our house to head to our local patch, Kilduff Farm in East Lothian. Surely the closest thing to Autumn magic you can get as a grown-up.

Slow Samhain Sundays

At this time of year, I try having slow Sunday mornings to top up my energy levels for the week ahead. After reading my book in bed, I love nothing more than a morning pottering in the kitchen. All year round is porridge season in our house, but the Autumn months are when I hear its comforting call most keenly. One of my favourite Autumn toppings is honey-roasted figs: chop three ripe figs into slices, drizzle with clear honey and top with a few dots of butter and a sprinkling of flaked almonds, then roast in the oven for 20 minutes at 200°C/Fan 180°C/Gas Mark 6. Meanwhile, soak your porridge in milk for at least 30 minutes, then cook low and slow with a generous pinch of sea salt until it slowly bubbles. Top with the cooked fruit and toasted nuts, including a drizzle of the juices. Autumn comfort in a bowl.

Hedgerow Harvest

Hedgerow bounty reaches its prime, often even better after the first frosts, which intensify the sugars. This is the perfect moment to make Christmas tipples to allow the fruit sufficient time to stew before December gift giving and imbibing. We collect sloes sparingly at our local nature reserve, but if you can't forage them, you can usually find sloes at farmers' markets and even online. Gran's best friend, Nan, used to make a dangerously drinkable sloe gin; her family recipe is a 3:2:1 ratio of sloes: caster sugar: gin. Leave for 6–8 weeks, shaking the bottle once a day for the first week. It tastes even better after a year or two left to stew. For non-drinkers like me, there's hedgerow jelly, tasty slathered on toast and deliciously adaptable. Combine an equal weight of hedgerow fruit and apples, chopped but not cored, in a big pan. Cook down with a little water until soft. Extract the juice overnight by straining the mixture through a muslin. The next day, add an equal amount of sugar to the juice and dissolve the mixture over a low heat, then boil until setting point is reached (see page 30). Decant into warm sterilised jars for a taste of Autumn over the colder months.

Visit an Orchard

Find a local community orchard or a pick-your-own farm and plan an afternoon of apple picking. Orchards are such biodiverse spaces, so why not take a sketchbook and sit for a wee while, sketching the trees and the wildlife you see? When you get home, if you're anything like me, you will have more apples than you know what to do with. After weeks of crumble (my family recipe is: 75g butter, 75g demerara sugar, 125g plain flour and 25g desiccated coconut rubbed together, sprinkled on top of 500g fruit and baked for 30 minutes at 210°C/Fan 190°C/Gas Mark 6), apple crisps are an easy and delicious way to preserve your haul. Simply peel and core them, finely slice, then thread them through a string or a long piece of dowelling and leave to dry out, undisturbed, for a few days.

PUMPKIN SEASON

The pumpkin has an interesting and varied history with links to British and Irish folklore. The carved 'Jack-O'-Lantern' is an Irish tradition; long before we decorated with pumpkins, the Irish carved turnips. The source of the name is an Irish folktale about a man called Stingy Jack who tricked the devil out of money. According to the tale, when Jack died God wouldn't let him into heaven and the devil wouldn't let him into hell, so he was doomed to walk the earth for all eternity. Afraid of Jack's return at Halloween, with the veil between worlds its thinnest, the Irish carved spooky expressions into turnips to scare off his tortured soul. Hence the two traditions became entwined. Subsequently, Irish immigrants brought the tradition across the pond, where the pumpkin was native to the region and – larger and thankfully easier to carve – was used as an alternative to the turnip. Thus, the pumpkin soon became a key part of Halloween decorations and celebrations.

When I was growing up, I remember Mum bravely carved 'neeps' or turnips (or swedes – it depends who you ask) which needed brute force and determination to decorate. Luckily, these days pumpkins are easy to come by around Samhain: seasonal, beautiful and delicious – as well as easier to carve.

SOURCING PUMPKINS

After World War II, the popularity of Halloween increased, and commercial pumpkin patches began to appear. A relatively minor crop until then, they were cultivated for this seasonal demand. These days, you can find pick-your-own pumpkin farms – a quick search online will alert you to your nearest patch. There is something magical about this Autumn tradition that can reconnect us with nature and our local farmers. Find out where your nearest is and support your local grower.

If there's no pumpkin patch near you, then your local farmers' market is sure to have a whole host of seasonal culinary pumpkins. If you're anything like me, you'll be like a kid in a sweetshop! I adore the 'Crown Prince' variety for its silvery blue skin and unexpectedly bright, yellow flesh, and they taste amazing roasted with the skin on. The miniature pumpkins such as 'Jill be Little' are lovely to eat (roast them whole and scoop out the seeds) and a great size to use as decorations until then. Pumpkins shouldn't be eye wateringly expensive, and make sure you actually want to eat them afterwards to get real value for money and avoid waste!

DECORATING IDEAS

In order to get the most out of your pumpkins, you need to keep them in the cool and away from any moisture. They look lovely by a fireplace or on the doorstep, but be sure to move them to somewhere sheltered, cool and dark if you want to eat them later. I've seen a big explosion in 'more is more' pumpkin decorating online but who can seriously eat that much pumpkin soup?! Stick to sizes and varieties you wish to eat. Ask yourself, do you really need so many, and will you definitely eat them all? Be honest!

I like to spend a while picking the prettiest pumpkins, as I like to let their natural beauty sing. If you're keen to carve it, choose a pumpkin with a smooth, rounded surface. In recent years, more abstract carving designs have become fashionable, such as repeated dots or holes (punched through with a drill bit). There's so much inspiration online, from simple yet effective designs to more complex and artistic ones.

I like to decorate my mantel using gourds (when the stove is not in use). I find arranging the pumpkins with the biggest in the middle is pleasing to the eye. Candles and fairy lights dotted between or inside them are a must. I've even seen some people carve their pumpkins and fill them with candle wax (such as beeswax) to make a seasonal tealight.

If you know you're not going to eat your gourds, or maybe they've become too hard to cut (as happens over time), you could paint them. Metallic paint (source an environmentally friendly one) can create a lovely lustrous finish, and copper is beautiful for transitioning your decorations into Yule. Graphic patterns in white paint, made using a chalkboard pen, work with a more minimal scheme. The possibilities are endless.

ZERO WASTE

Post-Halloween waste makes me sad. Once the holiday is over, many pumpkins are woefully neglected, however, there's no need for this – they keep for many months if stored in a cool, dry place, and there's so much you can make with them long into Winter.

What's great is that for some varieties you can use the whole squash. Use the peel to make crisps: sprinkle with olive oil, chilli flakes and sea salt and roast in the oven at 180°C/Fan 160°C/Gas Mark 4 for 20 minutes or so. Some varieties are tastier roasted whole with the skin on, as it helps them hold their shape and adds a contrasting textural dimension, so check before peeling.

You can also use the seeds: soak them in a bowl of cold water, then drain, dry and toast in a pan with spices and a little syrup for a sweet snack.

Once you're completely pumpkined-out, or if you have any that are well past their best, consider how to dispose of your gourd. Pets such as cats and dogs can eat pumpkin in moderation, or you could leave it in the garden for passing furry visitors – according to the RSPCA, birds, squirrels, badgers and foxes will all love it, as will farm animals such as pigs and chickens. Make sure to remove any tealights or wax if you've lit one as a lantern. However, if your pumpkin is mouldy, it could make animals sick, in which case you should put your pumpkin in the food waste or compost bin.

PUMPKIN FEAST

Samhain is the season we want to hunker down and get cosy in the kitchen. Whether you're hosting for a big group of friends or simply making your meal extra special for close family, it's well worth the effort to elevate the everyday.

Late Autumn is a time associated with gratitude and giving thanks. Although most strongly linked to America and Canada – a development from English Protestant harvest celebrations – many countries from Germany to Japan have variations on this theme as the year draws to a close. Modern-day Halloween celebrations have their roots in the Celtic festival Samhain, giving thanks to the end of Summer and marking the Celtic new year on 1 November. People believed that the souls of the dead would return to visit their families, and that those who died that year travelled to the next world. Catholic All Saints' Day took place on the same day, with All Hallows' Eve on 31 October, and then evolved into the Halloween we know.

Get back to the original meaning of these seasonal holidays by hosting a Samhain feast with good food, good company and gratitude. Identify the things you're grateful for – big or small – to ground you at this busy time and plan a Samhain celebration at home. It's the perfect excuse to set the table, light the candles, get out your best linens and gather together. Head out for a walk in the cold and return to a candlelit feast.

Eating seasonally is a way of connecting ourselves with the earth and cooking dark, real, seasonal foods offers comfort like nothing else. Here are some of my go-to gourd recipes for a Samhain celebration.

SPICED BUTTERNUT SQUASH SOUP

The sweetness of the squash is tempered by the heat from the chilli and sourness of tamarind, balanced by the fragrant and cooling coconut milk. Serve small portions as a starter or if you want to make this the main course, serve with generous hunks of sourdough bread and butter, and top with the squash peel crisps (see page 157) or toasted nuts and seeds.

SERVES 6

- 1 kg butternut squash or pumpkin, peeled and cubed
- 1 chilli, deseeded and chopped
- Approx. 1 tbsp olive oil
- 500ml vegetable stock, plus more if needed
- 400ml tin coconut milk
- 1 tbsp tamarind paste
- Sea salt and black pepper

Fry the squash and chilli in the olive oil in a large pan over a medium heat for about 15 minutes until starting to colour. Add the stock, bring to the boil and cook for about 20 minutes, or until soft.

Add the coconut milk and tamarind paste and heat through. Blend with a hand blender and loosen by stirring in more stock, if needed. Season with salt and pepper to taste, then serve.

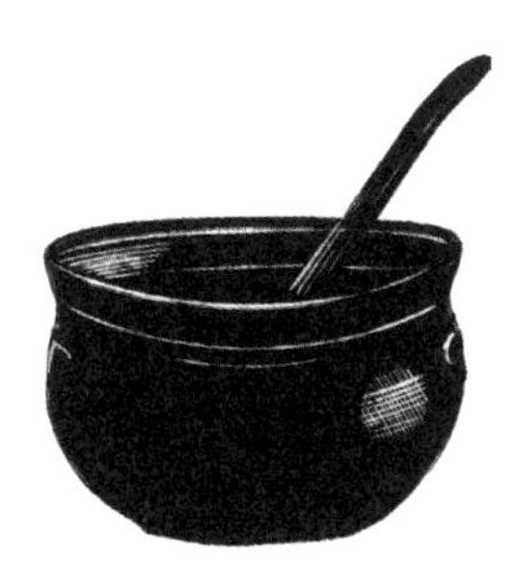

PUMPKIN & ROOT VEGETABLE CHILLI

A hearty veggie chilli makes for an easy but delicious sharing feast as you can easily scale the recipe up or down and you can serve it up in so many different ways: with a cornbread topping, with jacket potatoes, with mashed potato on top and browned under the grill, in tortilla wraps... Customise your chilli with whatever tins you have in the larder, swap in some soaked bulgur wheat or giant couscous and include your favourite pulses or vegetables. This chilli happens to be vegan too. I like to make the chilli the day before to leave its flavours to develop even more overnight, then simply warm through until bubbling and piping hot, and prepare whatever you're serving with it.

SERVES APPROX. 6

- 900g mixed pumpkin or butternut squash and sweet potato, peeled and cut into bite-sized chunks
- 2 tbsp olive oil, plus extra for drizzling
- 2 red onions, peeled and diced
- 1½ tsp paprika
- 3 tsp ground coriander
- 3 tsp ground cumin
- 2 tsp ground cinnamon
- 400g tin chickpeas, drained and rinsed
- 400g tin black beans
- 2 x 400g tins chopped tomatoes
- 250ml vegetable stock
- Sea salt and black pepper

Pre-heat the oven to 220°C/Fan 200°C/Gas Mark 7.

Drizzle the chunks of squash or pumpkin and sweet potato with olive oil and a sprinkling of salt, then roast for 30 minutes, until starting to brown.

Heat the 2 tablespoons of olive oil in a very large, heavy-based saucepan over a medium heat, add the onions and fry for 10 minutes or so, until translucent and caramelised.

Add the spices to the onions and stir for 2 minutes to cook them out and remove their bitterness.

Add the root vegetables to the pan, and stir to coat them in the spices, then tip in the pulses, chopped tomatoes and stock – enough to cover everything. Season to taste and raise the temperature. Bring to the boil, then simmer until the sauce has reduced and everything is tender – around 45 minutes in a large pan.

Season again if needed, then serve.

CHOCOLATE CAKE WITH PUMPKIN CURD & SPICED CHOCOLATE BUTTERCREAM

Chocolate and pumpkin go surprisingly well together: here the sponge is sandwiched with a sweet spiced buttercream and zesty pumpkin curd.

To make your own pumpkin purée: chop pumpkin flesh into 2cm chunks and boil or steam it for about 15 minutes until tender, then blend to a loose consistency.

SERVES 6–8

Chocolate cake
- 100g butter
- 225g caster sugar
- 2 large free-range eggs
- 200g self-raising flour
- 2 tbsp cocoa powder
- Pinch of sea salt
- 150ml milk

Pumpkin curd
- 100g pumpkin purée (tinned, or see intro)
- 50g caster sugar
- Zest and juice of 1 clementine (about 50ml juice)
- 50g butter
- 1 free-range egg

Spiced chocolate buttercream
- 60g butter
- 250g icing sugar
- 2 tbsp warm milk
- 1 tbsp cocoa powder
- ½ tsp cinnamon
- ¼ tsp mixed spice
- ¼ tsp cardamom

Pre-heat the oven to 180°C/Fan 160°C/Gas Mark 4. Grease and line two cake tins.

Cream the butter and sugar in a mixing bowl until light and fluffy, then beat in the eggs, one at a time, with a little flour. Fold in the rest of the flour along with the cocoa powder and sea salt and loosen with the milk.

Pour into the prepared tins and bake for 30 minutes, or until a skewer placed in the centre of the cakes comes out clean. Remove from the tins and leave to cool on a wire rack.

In a pan over a low heat, mix the pumpkin purée with the sugar, clementine zest and juice and stir until the sugar dissolves.

Add the butter to the warm mixture and stir it through until it melts. Turn the heat down to the lowest setting. Add the egg and stir the mixture continuously over a low heat for about 15 minutes, or until the mixture thickens and coats the back of a spoon.

Decant the curd into a bowl and cover loosely with cling film (to stop a skin forming). Pop in the fridge and leave to firm up for at least 30 minutes.

Meanwhile, make the buttercream by beating the butter, icing sugar and milk for about 5 minutes until light and airy, and almost white in colour. Add the cocoa powder and spices and give them a good mix.

Once cooled, cover one of the cakes with half the buttercream. Fill with about 4 tablespoons of the curd and spread (there will be some leftover – delicious on toast).

Sandwich the other cake on top and add the rest of the buttercream, spreading it evenly over the top. Decorate with more pumpkin curd and serve.

Seasonal Celebrations of Nature

There's something enchanting about being outside as the golden days peak then fade into Winter. Stormy nights and gales act as a catalyst for the rapidly approaching colder days, while longer nights trigger nature's hibernation, leading to behaviour changes and spectacular late Autumn sights.

The trees continue to turn shades of red and gold, and if the weather is particularly dry, the colours seem even more vibrant. Broad-leaf trees are most spectacular. Rowan berries are abundant and their leaves turn from green to russet and saffron hues. Some trees – such as the oak – wait until November to show their spectacular colours to the world. And by the end of the month most branches have lost their leaves until the Spring.

In the forest, evergreen mosses are now visible, their emerald tufts bright against the stark bare wood and spongey underfoot. Berries still abound. In late Autumn sweet chestnuts ripen and fall. Concealed in spiky cases, they are worth the effort to gather – either freeze ready for Winter or roast and eat straight away. Fungi are at their height in October. Foraging them is advisable only if you really know what you're doing but spotting them can be just as fun.

Animals are preparing for the tough months ahead. As the land becomes increasingly bare, hares (who, unlike their rabbit friends, do not burrow) can be seen crouching in the undergrowth. Spiders' webs adorn the countryside, stunning sights following heavy dew or frosts. By now, the squirrels will have beaten you to acorns and conkers if you weren't quick enough, and hedgehogs are collecting leaves and bracken to make their nests ready for hibernation. Check for them beneath piles of leaves, particularly if you're making a bonfire.

Keep an eye out for deer in woodlands and in the countryside; though they can be a challenge to spot, you will probably hear them before you see them as males noisily compete for female attention. Hedgehogs, dormice and bats are the main species that hibernate in the UK, reducing their metabolism and living off fat reserves throughout Winter. It's good to neglect the garden a little to provide them raw material for nesting (as good an excuse as any). Left to their own devices, many plants dry out, providing valuable food for birds and important habitats for insects.

If you hear an unmissable honking overhead and see a tell-tale V-shape in the sky then you've been witness to the spectacular flight of geese. From Siberia, mud-loving Brent geese take shelter in our estuaries while Barnacle geese prefer north-western climes. Starling murmurations are surely one of the most stunning Autumn wildlife spectacles and peak from November into early December. Starlings arrive in their hundreds of thousands, moving in huge groups that rise and fall in perfect synchronisation; at first glance they appear as a cloud. Starlings are best seen during the early evening when they head to their shelters for the night.

Falling leaves reveal bare branches and berries: a potential feast to smaller species such as finches and blue tits. You can view migrating birds, including wading birds on wetlands and islands, at local wildlife reserves and protected sites – they tend to stick to the coasts on their defined routes. Search for local observatories and be sure to check the tides; high tides bring the birds closer to shore.

Look for grey seals on the coast's quiet coves and beaches; in the Autumn they congregate en masse at certain on shore sites to mate. Their young are born and nursed on the shore; try to spot the tiny white pups but don't disturb them.

Atlantic salmon return to rivers to spawn, battling currents, waterfalls and other hazards through the rivers swollen with Autumn rains to return to the very place they were born, so focused on their mission they don't even feed. Those who do make it pair up in shallow spawning grounds where, once mated, they die. Early mornings or evenings are the best times to try to spot them, especially after rain.

COLLECTING & CRAFTING WITH PINE CONES

Even after the leaves have fallen, I find there's a surprising amount to see. This is the conifers' time to shine! Pine cones mostly fall to the ground between September and December, peaking around Samhain. You can find them scattered beneath pine trees in gardens, woodlands and parks in city and country alike.

Hunting for pine cones is an activity steeped in nostalgia for me, and finding them is just as much fun as decorating with them. In the Autumn and Winter I often find my pockets filled with pine cones, a habit that dates back to childhood. Months after Winter, I still find random pine cones that I just couldn't leave behind surfacing in handbags or hiding at the bottom of baskets.

My favourite place to find pine cones now is Dawyck Botanical Gardens in the Scottish Borders, which has a mind-bogglingly tall collection of native and non-native pine trees. I adore the distinctive shape of the Douglas Fir and the many miniature cones of larch, often festooned with furry lichens and mosses.

Pine cones are actually the fruit of the pine tree, used for reproduction – the scales of the cone keep the seeds hidden beneath safe and warm until it's time to be released into the ground and make future trees. As such, in folklore pines and firs represent fertility, good fortune and even protection. Over the years – and poring over my vintage *Observer's Books* collection – I've come to identify different types of pine and their cones. Here are a few favourites; please remember to gather responsibly – a few from each area that have fallen naturally to the ground will be more than sufficient.

COMMON PINE TREES

Scots pine
(*Pinus sylvestris*)

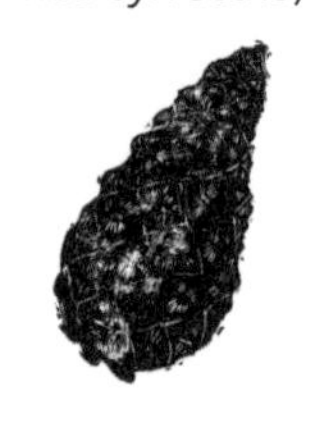

The Scots pine is one of only three conifers native to the UK and our only native species of pine. Perhaps unsurprisingly given its name, it is the national tree of Scotland – and often home to rare Scottish wildlife including the red squirrel, capercaillie and wildcats. It has reddish-brown bark, fading to a darker shade at the bottom and blue-green, slightly twisted needles. Scots pine cones mature slowly, so every year there is a mix of new and old cones – the fallen, mature cones are a greyish-brown with a raised bump on top of each scale.

Larch
(*Larix decidua*)

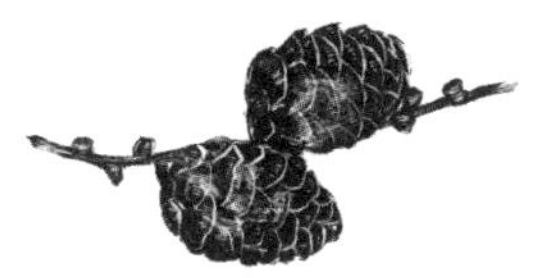

The larch is unusual in that it is a deciduous pine tree. It is friend to squirrels, birds and moths alike. You will notice the amber, needle-like leaves of the larch falling in the Autumn, leaving behind pinkish-brown branches filled with masses of small oval cones. In folklore the larch is believed to protect against enchantment and evil spirits so was historically worn or burnt. As its branches are light and numerous, you can often find them fallen after storms – their sculptural shape looks beautiful in a vase.

Douglas fir
(*Pseudotsuga menziesii*)

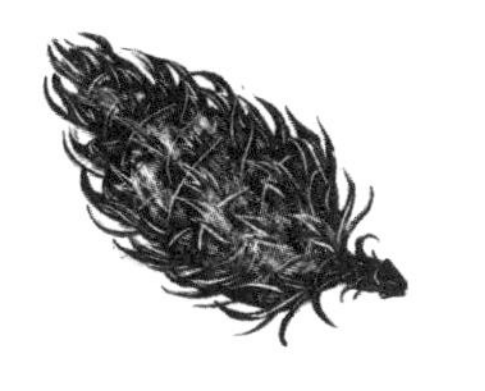

This non-native pine was brought to the UK from America in the 1800s by David Douglas and can live for up to 1,000 years. It grows to over fifty metres tall, making it an ideal height for birds of prey. Its needles are flat and distributed around the twigs, with a white stripe underneath. Douglas fir cones hang straight down from the branches with three points emerging from each scale. It is probably best known as a variety of Christmas tree.

Black pine
(*Pinus negra*)

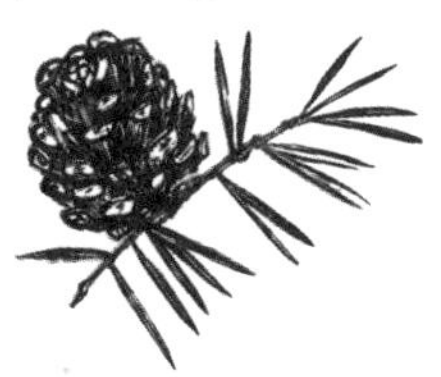

The black pine is triangular in shape when young, has dense branches and a grey-brown bark. It has pairs of long pine needles, up to fifteen centimetres long, and large cones up to eight centimetres long with prickled scales. It is a popular ornamental and commercial tree as it grows quickly and is often used in paper manufacture and construction. In the wild, the black pine offers shelter to birds and even deer.

Norway spruce
(*Picea abies*)

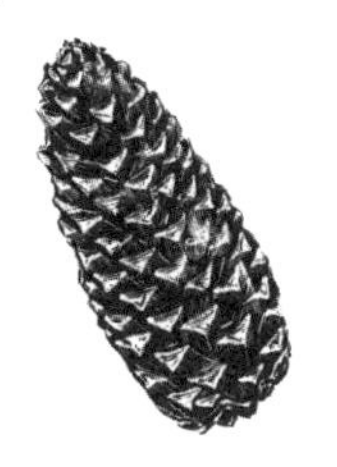

This European tree, native to Scandinavia, was first popularised by Prince Albert and is now synonymous with the festive season. It is tall, straight and triangular in appearance – making it ideal for decorating – and its square, pointed needles emit a rich, sweet fragrance. The Norway spruce also has long pine cones that hang down, with overlapping scales and pointed tips.

PINE CONE GARLAND

Pine cones always featured in my seasonal decorating growing up – lined up on the mantel, or placed generously in bowls, then later hung on the tree. When I was younger, glitter was definitely one of my favourite things in my craft box. These days, we know that it often contains microplastics, which are harmful to the environment, but luckily for fans of the sparkle there are many different eco-friendly glitters on the market now. Just as well, really, as I think we need all the sparkle that we can get. Of course, you could make this garland without the glitter but I think it adds a little something extra special.

YOU WILL NEED

- Old cloth or newspapers
- Pine cones in varying sizes (or other natural materials, such as acorns or alder cones)
- 2 small paint brushes
- Craft glue
- Eco-friendly glitter
- Natural twine
- Scissors
- Miniature bells, ribbons or other decorations (optional)

Start by covering your table or work surface with a cloth or something to protect your furniture, so that you can use this to save, gather and reuse excess glitter.

Using a small brush, dab the tips of a pine cone with a thin layer of craft glue (less is more).

Decant a little glitter into a small bowl, then dip the pine cone into the glitter and tap to get rid of the excess. Continue, adding glitter to some more (or all!) of the pine cones. Repeat with your other natural materials, if using: experiment, covering all or part of them in glitter and leaving some plain.

Leave the glue to dry, after which time the pine cones will probably need another wee shake or dry brush (with the clean paintbrush) to get rid of stray glitter – although it's all part of that homemade charm.

To start assembling the garland, measure the space you want the garland to cover, then add a little extra to accommodate the knots for hanging the garland, and then cut your twine to size.

Create a loop on one end and firmly knot it. You could even cover the knot with a tightly tied bell or a ribbon.

Next, simply tie the pine cones to the twine underneath their scales as close as you can to the top – or on their stems if they have them. I like to alternate different styles of decorated or plain pine cones, spacing them evenly along the length of the twine.

Once you're almost at the end of your twine, make a loop at the other end, tie on the last bell or ribbon to cover the knot, and then position your garland wherever you want to decorate.

PINE SUGAR SHORTBREAD

Pine can be foraged and infused in baking; it has a citrus, aromatic, almost herbal flavour. Each pine has a slightly different flavour too: Douglas fir is the most complex, while larch is delicious picked early in the Spring and preserved in a pine sugar or syrup for bakes when its needles are pale green. Just make sure you identify your pines carefully and avoid yew, which is toxic to humans and animals – it has straight, short needles with pointed tips, dark green on top and grey-green below, with red, berry-like structures.

I like to make pine sugar, which becomes more flavourful the longer you leave it to infuse. This is not an exact science, and very much depends how 'piney' you like things. Experiment and see how strong you like the flavour. The further ahead you prepare the pine sugar, the longer the flavours will have to develop, so keep that in mind, too.

A pine sugar shortbread is perfect to celebrate the Scottish Patron saint on St Andrew's Day at the end of November. My family's traditional shortbread recipe uses the standard 1:2:3 ratio of sugar: butter: flour.

MAKES APPROX. 24 (DEPENDING ON THE SIZE OF YOUR CUTTER)

For the Douglas fir sugar

250g caster sugar
Handful of Douglas fir needles, brown ends trimmed

For the shortbread

150g plain flour
100g butter, cubed
50g Douglas fir sugar, plus extra for dusting

I always make more Douglas fir sugar than I need, to use in the coming months: in a blender whizz together the sugar and needles until the needles have begun to break down and release their oils.

You should be left with a fine, green-tinged sugar flecked with bits. If you want to use the sugar straight away, sift the sugar to get rid of the tough, stringy parts of the needles. Otherwise you can leave the pine needles in the sugar, stored in an airtight container, to infuse for longer until you want to bake with it.

To make the shortbread, place the flour and butter in a large bowl and rub together lightly with the tips of your fingers to form a crumb-like texture. Add the Douglas fir sugar and mix with your hands, squishing it together (technical term) to form a dough.

Chill the dough in the fridge for 30 minutes. Towards the end of this time, pre-heat the oven to 180°C/Fan 160°C/Gas Mark 4 and line a baking tray with greaseproof paper.

Roll out the dough until 2–3mm thick. Using a small cutter, cut out shapes and place them on the lined baking tray, leaving a little space between each – they will expand, but only a wee bit.

Bake for 10–12 minutes until golden.

Sprinkle with more Douglas fir sugar while still warm, then leave to cool and firm up. The shortbread will keep for up to 1 week in an airtight container – if it lasts that long.

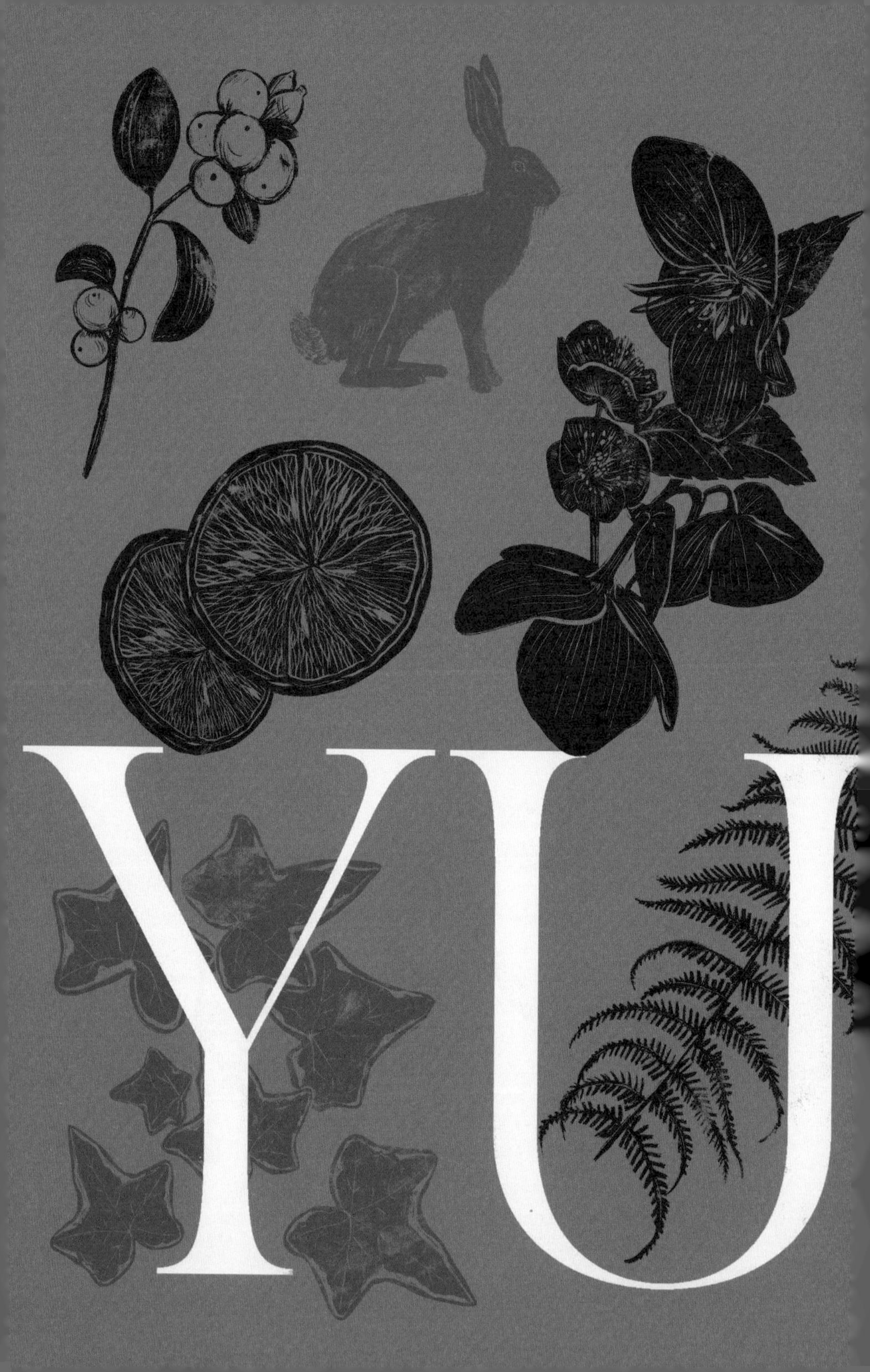
YU

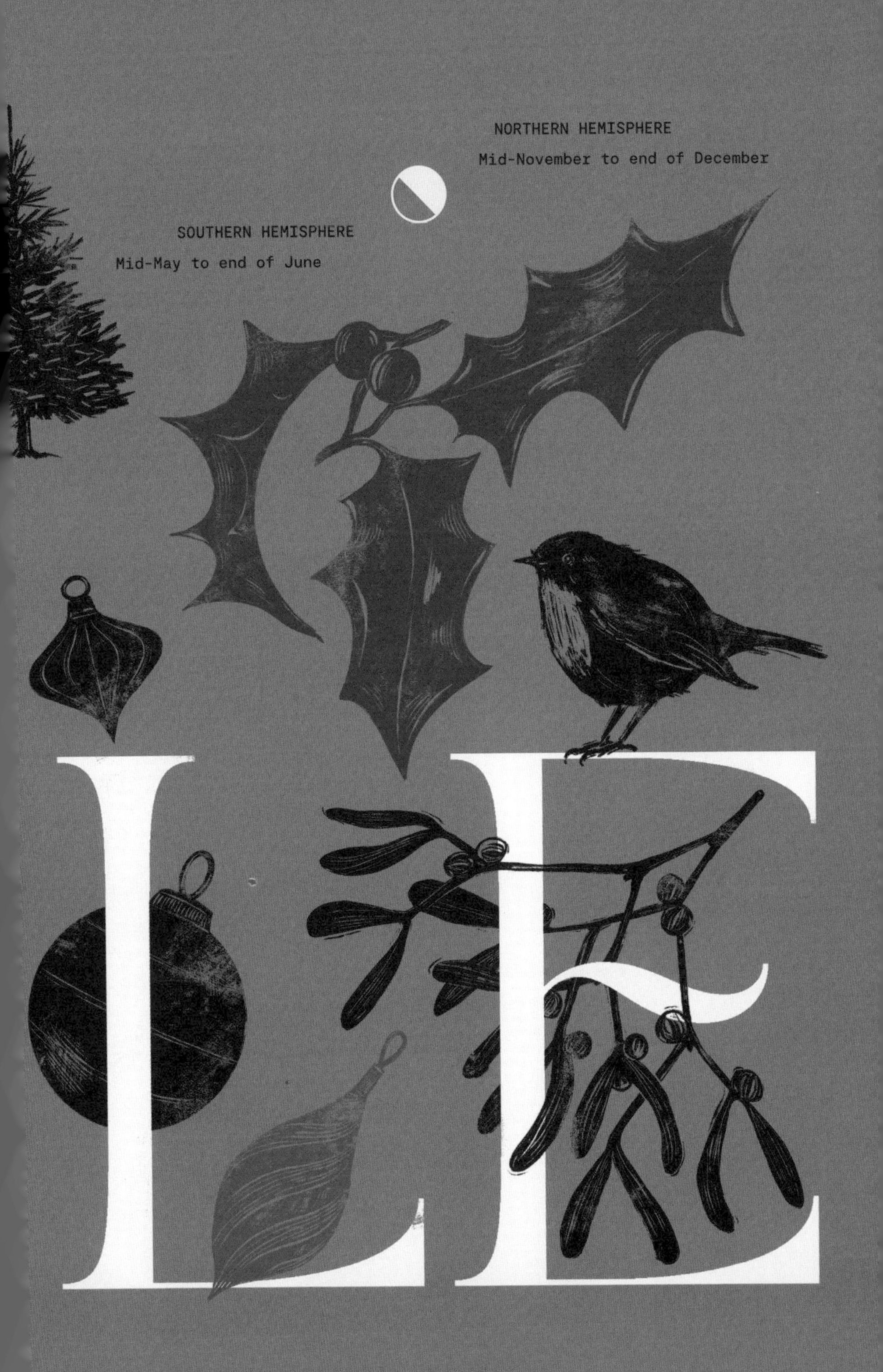
NORTHERN HEMISPHERE
Mid-November to end of December
SOUTHERN HEMISPHERE
Mid-May to end of June
LE

MIDWINTER MAGIC

Yule. The darkest days of the year should be a time for slowing down, reflection and quiet. Yet too often we're under even more pressure than usual to seek perfection: the perfect gifts, the perfect host, the perfect Christmas lunch. At the same time, we feel anxious not to miss out, to say yes to every invite, to forget our boundaries. Christmas adverts and social media marketing urge us ever onwards to consume, consume, consume.

It's no wonder that it can all feel like a bit much. This year, I encourage you to take things gradually, to take stock and to practise saying no. To step back from the frantic festive preparations. To stop for a moment and appreciate the magic of Midwinter. To simplify. To sparkle. To embrace home and hearth to get back to the true meaning of Yule.

In the Celtic Wheel of the Year, Yule coincides with the longest night as darkness reaches its peak at the Winter Solstice. For a few days, the sun rises at around the same time before rising a few minutes earlier each day. We are in the depths of Winter, but the Wheel keeps turning and the light slowly begins to return. This is a simultaneous ending and beginning as the year draws to its dark close, and the new year is born.

Many modern-day festive celebrations have their roots in pre-Christian traditions, the lines between Yule and Christmas becoming blurred. One thing they have in common is the focus on fire and feasting. Simple, seasonal fare and good company are the only ingredients you need – you don't have to have a perfect meal or day.

Yule for me is the epitome of homemade celebration, where the joy is found in the making: from what we gift, to everything we eat, to the decorations I bring out year after year. I have fond memories of making salt dough with Mum and she still brings the same decorations out of the Christmas box, complete with tiny fingerprints, every festive season. Mum's fudge recipe is one I learnt by watching and now make and gift to friends and family.

Another favourite part of each season in the Celtic Wheel is decorating, inspired always by nature. During Yule I take my cues from the Celts and their evergreen simplicity, with its symbolism of life and longevity. As Christmas was banned in Scotland for centuries, historically the decorations weren't put up until just a few days before Christmas, which I'm mindful of today: decorating slowly, simply, enjoying the process and the delayed gratification this brings.

It's easy to get swept up in the pre-Christmas hysteria, but before you throw yourself into preparations, try to take stock of your own needs.

SAVOUR THE QUIET MYSTERY OF MIDWINTER AS THE NIGHTS DRAW OUT AGAIN.

Seasonal Celebrations at Home

The best part of the festive season, for me, has always been the anticipation. There's so much more to Christmas than Christmas Day, and I think the Celts had it right by revelling in the build-up and aftermath of Yule during the darkest months of the year. The pinnacle of the season – the Winter Solstice – or the longest night and shortest day (usually around 21 December) is a quiet but special time that is often overlooked in favour of the 'big days' of the Christian holidays, but I've been heartened to see others celebrating Midwinter as well as Christmas in recent years. Whatever you believe, these dark days are a time where we need magic, creativity, slowness and gentle celebration as an antidote to the louder, busier festive season and call to consume that has more recently evolved.

Pay it Forward

If, like me, you enjoy the countdown as much as the height of celebratory days, then a personalised 'Advent' calendar (mine counts down to Yule) made up of experiences involving giving as well as receiving will bring even more Yuletide joy. You could source some miniature drawers (I found some mid-century tool drawers waiting for me in a vintage shop), hang envelopes from a branch with ribbons, or buy or make a wall hanging with pockets. The most important thing is the thought put into your daily prompts. You might want to include a mixture of experiences and things to look forward to – trips to a Christmas fair, to visit a relative or to see the local ballet production – and opportunities to reflect or give back: a prompt to practise gratitude, to donate produce to the local foodbank, or to volunteer with a local charity. This way, you focus on making memories and sharing the special parts of the season with others. And a chocolate coin slipped in with each prompt always helps.

Festive Fudge

I've always made treats for my family and friends, and it's now so much a part of my own Christmas build-up that I dare say I enjoy the ritual just as much as the recipient. In recent years I've adapted a favourite family fudge recipe to make and gift my own festive spiced version. It is easier to make than you think – just be careful, as the sugar gets incredibly hot. This recipe makes enough to fill four 250ml jars: mix 500g caster sugar, a 397g can of condensed milk and 100g butter in a medium-sized, heavy-based saucepan over a gentle heat. While the mixture melts together, grease and line a 20cm square baking tray with greaseproof paper and fill the sink with 5cm cold water. Once the sugar has dissolved, increase the heat to bring the fudge mixture to the boil, stirring frequently so that it doesn't burn, until it turns caramel coloured, thickens and reaches 112°C on a sugar thermometer. (This is called 'soft ball stage'. You could also fill a shallow dish with cold water, drop a little mixture into it, then remove it: if ready, the fudge should form together into a ball in your fingers, setting immediately.) This should take around 15 minutes. Remove from the heat and add the zest of ½ lemon and 1 clementine along with ½ teaspoon ground cinnamon and ½ teaspoon ground mixed spice and a pinch of crushed sea salt flakes. Stir until thoroughly combined. Quickly dunk the pan in the sink of cold water (do not get any water in the fudge). Beat the mixture as it cools and thickens, and becomes grainy as it begins to set. Pour into the prepared tin and mark squares on the top once it has cooled a little. Wait until completely cold before cutting the fudge into bite-sized pieces.

Chocolate Treats

Chocolate is a failsafe gift and I like to have a stash ready for last-minute presents over the festive season. Mendiants are incredibly easy to make and always go down well. These traditional Christmastime French chocolates can be decorated with whichever nuts and fruits you have in the larder. Be as creative as you like: dried cranberries, crystallised ginger and toasted pistachios are particularly festive. Grease and line a baking tray with greaseproof paper. Finely chop your desired topping – for every 100g of chocolate, you need around a tablespoon of topping. Chop the chocolate into small pieces and place in a heatproof bowl. Fill a small saucepan with a few centimetres of water and bring to the boil. Set the small bowl on top (make sure the bottom doesn't touch the water) and leave the chocolate until it is half melted – don't stir yet. Set aside to let the residual heat finish melting the chocolate, then stir until smooth and glossy. Spoon the chocolate onto the tray in small circles and sprinkle with the topping, working quickly before the chocolate solidifies. It's best to make your mendiants in small batches, decorating as you go, so you can re-melt the chocolate if you need to. Leave to cool and set – avoid putting the chocolate in the fridge as it will lose its sheen and take on a dusty bloom – then peel away the mendiants and present in your desired container.

Christmas Books

Growing up, we had a Christmas 'book box' where our favourite festive reads were stored; personal highlights included *Maisie's Merry Christmas* and *The Jolly Christmas Postman* as well as traditional tales such as *The Nutcracker*. I have fond memories of Mum getting the box down from the attic when we were wee, the books being even more special for their rare outing. These days I have started my own Christmas book collection and seasonal reading traditions. My favourites include Jeanette Winterson's *Christmas Days* and *Little Women*. I bring out seasonal cookbooks such as *Christmas at River Cottage* by Lucy Brazier and Nigel Slater's *The Christmas Chronicles* so I can revel in their recipes and inspiration for these few, precious weeks. Gifting books at Christmas is another, much-loved family tradition – the comforting lull between Christmas and Hogmanay is usually spent curled up with a new book.

Gift Wrapping

In the run-up to Yule the diary can fill up quickly with social obligations. This year, set your own boundaries and don't say yes to everything. If a particular social situation fills you with dread, question why that is and consider re-prioritising. There's so much pressure to be busy, busy, busy, but if you hate the local Christmas market because you can't move for people, don't force yourself to go. And once you've made the decision don't dwell on it. In recent years, I've found that doing fewer things means that I can slow down and enjoy the tasks that usually get pushed to the last minute.

Gift wrapping, for instance. Rather than fussing with lots of bags and fancy wrapping, keeping it simple with recycled brown paper tied with leftover ribbon (saved from candles, cakes, anything) and decorated with a piece of foliage or dried flowers (perhaps offcuts from wreath making) is simple and chic. If you want to personalise your wrapping, you could use stamps – I have some cherished ones from childhood, and some more recent ones with woodland motifs. You could even make your own stamps by carving potatoes into simple shapes: halve a small potato across the middle, then dry the exposed ends with a tea towel. Press a small cookie cutter into the cut end of the potato – just enough to create a guide – then cut round the cutter with a sharp knife to make your stamp. Repeat with a different stamp on the other half of the potato. Firmly press your stamp onto an ink pad and stamp the whole of the paper before you wrap – it's usually easier to go with a random pattern than neat rows. Clean the stamp carefully between each ink colour. I would advise making new potato stamps each year.

You could also swap paper for fabric, wrapping gifts with pretty tea towels, scarves or even fabric scraps. Look up Japanese furoshiki wrapping – an ancient, traditional way to store clothes and other objects. Essentially you wrap your gift in a square of fabric, tied with a bow, that can be loved and reused for many years to come. Thoughtful and beautiful.

CHOCOLATE & PEPPERMINT BUNDT CAKE

Making a Christmas cake is a lovely tradition, and it can make a thoughtful gift for bakers and non-bakers alike. This chocolate peppermint Bundt cake is perfect for those who aren't fans of the traditional fruitcake, with seasonal flavour and visual impact. The cake has a tender crumb and the peppermint chocolate ganache is festive and indulgent. You can get traditional shaped Bundt tins in baking shops and even supermarkets; it does make the cake look extra special, but you could bake this in a standard cake tin too.

SERVES 6–8

140g butter, plus extra, melted, for brushing
75g milk chocolate, chopped
35g cocoa powder
1 tsp peppermint extract
50ml boiling water
260g caster sugar
2 free-range eggs
200g self-raising flour
100ml Greek yoghurt

For the ganache
100ml double cream
50g mint chocolate, chopped

Pre-heat the oven to 170°C/Fan 150°C/Gas Mark 3½. Brush the inside of a Bundt tin generously with melted butter.

Place the milk chocolate in a bowl set over a pan of simmering water, making sure that the bottom of the bowl doesn't touch the water. Allow the chocolate to become half melted, then remove from the heat and allow the residual heat to do the rest of the melting.

Sift in the cocoa powder and add the peppermint extract and loosen with enough of the boiling water to make a thick paste. Set aside to cool.

Cream the butter and sugar with a wooden spoon until pale and fluffy. Add the eggs one at a time with a little of the flour, then stir in the yoghurt, followed by the chocolate paste.

Fold in the remaining flour, being careful not to over-mix. Pour into the prepared tin and smooth the surface.

Bake for 40–45 minutes (or 50–55 minutes if using a standard cake tin), until a skewer inserted in the middle comes out clean.

Leave to cool for at least 15 minutes, if not longer – and then turn out onto a wire rack to cool completely.

To make the ganache, heat the cream until it is just about to boil, then remove from the heat and add the chopped mint chocolate. Leave to stand and let the residual heat do the work, then stir until the chocolate has melted and the lumps disappear.

Pour over the cooled Bundt and leave to set, then serve.

SEASONAL CRAFTS

In our house, the decorations don't go up until just before Yule. Over the last few years, I've honed a small collection of decorations that really mean something to me – so their eventual unveiling is all the special for the anticipation.

Every piece has a story. When I left home, I started a tradition of buying only one, very special bauble each year – my first few were from Liberty London when I lived in the capital. This approach means gradually building a quality collection of special pieces you will love and cherish forever. Bringing these decorations out each year is like a portal to your past self.

Vintage and thrifted baubles are the most sustainable options. I was lucky enough to inherit a few, very special baubles from my grandparents: the traditional 1950s jewel hued glass creations are like nothing made today, and they're among my most special possessions. You can find similar traditional baubles at vintage fairs, though in some parts they can be on the pricey side. Set a budget and be ready to haggle!

Collecting aside, one of the things I relish most in the run-up to Christmas is making my own decorations. It's as much a part of my countdown to Yule as mince pies and Christmas music. In the busy festive season, setting aside a little time to craft is vital to help me slow down, get into creative flow and leave the seasonal to-do lists to one side – even for an hour or two.

Christmas decorations have been homemade for centuries. In medieval times, evergreen boughs were hung from the ceiling and decorated with seasonal fruit. Many of our most popular Christmas crafts today originate from the Victorians: from Christmas crackers to tree ornaments to wreaths. And, of course, the greenery comes from the Pagans – as I explore on pages 184–5.

No matter what the finished product looks like, it's the act of making itself – and making memories – that is most important. Here, I talk you through some simple crafts to try at home in just an hour or two.

SALT DOUGH DECORATIONS

This festive make fills me with the most nostalgia. The dough is made from three household ingredients and is so simple to make yet looks really effective, and can be customised into different designs and projects as well as easily scaled up or down. It's a great craft to do with little ones – I have cherished memories of making this at the kitchen table with Mum and my brother.

MAKES APPROX. 50 (DEPENDING ON THE SIZE OF YOUR CUTTER)

50g table salt
100g plain flour, plus extra for dusting
50ml water

You will need
Cookie cutters
Thin knitting needle
Twine or ribbon

In a large bowl with plenty of room to knead, thoroughly mix together the salt and flour.

Add the water and stir in with a spoon, then knead with your hands, pressing everything together until it starts to form a dough.

Transfer the dough to a lightly floured surface and continue to knead for a few more minutes until your dough is smooth and even. Line two baking trays with greaseproof paper.

Lightly re-flour the surface if needed, then roll out your dough evenly to around 3mm thick. Stamp out shapes in the dough with the cookie cutter, and place them on the trays spaced slightly apart.

Pre-heat the oven to its lowest setting while you re-roll your offcuts and then stamp out as many shapes as you can; repeat until the dough is all used up.

Use the pointy end of a knitting needle to poke a hole in the top of each shape so you can hang them or attach them to something once they've set. You could also mark patterns in the dough with the knitting needle or press objects into them – for instance baking stamps or natural finds such as pine cones. Experiment and see the textures you are drawn to.

Bake in the oven for 3 hours, or until solid. Halfway through, turn the shapes over so they cook evenly on both sides.

Leave to cool completely, then use as desired: decorate with paint, eco-friendly glitter, foraging finds or anything you have to hand. I like to leave them plain as I am drawn to the blank canvas of the porcelain white finish.

If hanging the salt dough shapes as decorations, measure out twice the length of the drop you want, plus 2cm. Cut the ribbon to size, then thread through and tie at the top with a double knot, or a bow if you're feeling fancy.

YULE CANDLE

Scottish and Scandinavian traditions involve burning a huge ornamental candle, often in festive shades of red and green or decorated with holly or other evergreens. As the timing of festive celebrations began to shift, the candle would be lit by the head of the household on Christmas Eve and burnt throughout the night – it was often thought to be bad luck if it burnt out before Christmas Day arrived. In Scotland, the candles were often given as gifts and would be placed at the table during Christmas Eve dinner. Decorating your own dinner candles adds a personalised touch to contemporary celebrations.

YOU WILL NEED

Plain, unscented wax dinner candles
Alcohol wet wipes
Old cloth or newspaper
Scrap paper
Candle holder (optional)
Small paint brush or sponge
Water-based, non-toxic acrylic paint (this is important – it must be water-based to be safe to burn)
Jar of water

First, wipe your candles down with the wet wipes to prepare their surfaces for painting, and then let them air dry.

Protect your work surface with paper or a cloth you don't mind getting paint on.

Plan out, experiment and practise your designs and colour palette on the scrap paper. This has to translate into three dimensions – so simple, repeat designs work best, as does a limited colour palette.

Once you're happy with your design, copy it onto the candle with a first coat of paint colour, going in with just a tiny bit of paint on your brush (you can layer up if you need more, but if it is too thick the paint will chip). Either decorate one side at a time, if you prefer painting flat, or pop the candle in the candle holder and turn it as you go. Don't worry about it being perfect – that's all part of the homemade charm!

Clean your brush in the water, then leave the paint to dry.

Go in with your next colour. Repeat, adding the smallest details last. If you mess up, don't worry – just wipe it off with the wet wipes, air dry and start again.

Leave your candles for a few hours until completely dry before you burn them.

Tips

- You can get wax pens for this job and even special kits, but I prefer to use what I have to hand, as I usually have multi-purpose paints for different crafts.
- Turn your Yule candle into an Advent candle by painting numbers down one side or spiralling them around the candle.

DRIED CITRUS

Scent is so evocative at Christmastime, and drying your own citrus fruits is a sure-fire way to make your home smell, and feel, festive. December marks the arrival of citrus fruits, just in time for festive baking and crafting. This is the perfect slow craft as so much of this make is hands off – time is what does the magic here. You can dry out all kinds of citrus fruits, so experiment and see what you find the most effective. Once they have dried out, you can use them to make all manner of decorations (see below).

YOU WILL NEED

1 large orange or 3 clementines, sliced 1cm thick

Pre-heat the oven to 110°C/Fan 100°C/Gas Mark ¼ and set a wire rack on top of a baking tray.

Press the orange slices between a couple of pieces of kitchen paper to remove excess moisture.

Place in a single layer on the wire rack – this will allow air to circulate around the whole fruit.

Bake for 45 minutes, then turn the citrus slices over and bake for another 45 minutes.

If they're still a little tacky, turn again and bake for another 15 minutes. Keep a close eye on them as they can burn. The timing will depend on your oven's own quirks.

Repeat until they are firm – the slices should feel dried out and have no moisture left.

Remove from the oven and allow to cool completely before storing in an airtight container. Use as desired.

Some ideas for what to make with your dried citrus slices

- Make a garland by threading twine through two points at the top of each citrus slice, so the twine passes behind the flesh.
- Thread twine through one point at the top of each slice, make a loop and tie, then hang on the Christmas tree. Position them in front of a fairy light so the light shines through.
- Attach to wrapped presents with a little twine, to decorate.
- Use ribbon to tie fruit slices around napkins on your table.
- Scatter slices over the table or mantelpiece.
- Use them to decorate wreaths and swags – for example, to make the Autumn Wreath on page 134 look wintry.

Seasonal Celebrations of Nature

The passage from Autumn to Winter is complete, seasonal storms rapidly removing the last leaves from the trees. If we're lucky, cold, crisp days where the light is ice clear and frost lingers are a regular occurrence, rather than the horizontal rain and gales that too often characterise a Scottish Winter. The branches are bare, but evergreens lift the dull, brown landscape of the Winter months. In the UK, while some animals are hibernating, plenty of wildlife can still be spotted as the natural surroundings are more exposed.

Evergreens shine. As well as the ubiquitous pine trees (see page 164–5), holly is the evergreen stereotypically associated with Yule. However, it is often stripped of its iconic red berries by the time it arrives, thanks to hungry birds! Larch trees have lost their amber needles by now, leaving behind bare branches with beautiful miniature cones. Snowberries are easy to spot, their bulbous white clumps of berries dancing on thin, now-bare branches, while clumps of evergreen mistletoe cling to trees, especially apple and oak, with instantly recognisable, dewy white berries and forked leaves.

Some flowers can still be found against Winter's predominant palette of brown and grey if you look carefully. My favourite Winter flowers, hellebores, begin to flower, the white Christmas rose arriving just in time for festive gifting and enjoyment. Winter heliotrope can be found in damp, shady areas, its heart-shaped leaves forming a carpet of greenery alongside textural ferns.

Animals such as squirrels are still busy gathering food for the long months ahead, making the most of the earlier evenings. Make sure you protect your Spring bulbs, or you might find garden visitors snacking on your precious tulips – chilli powder is said to deter squirrels. Despite our changing climate, some British species of wildlife turn white in Winter, once a tactic to camouflage themselves against snowy landscapes. Not the best strategy these days, but it does make them easier to spot – for instance, if you're walking quietly in the hills and see a flash of blueish-white, you're likely to have seen a mountain hare.

Bare branches can also help us to spot birds such as rooks and crows, which roost in woodlands. The short-eared owl hunts in the daytime (unlike the more famous barn or tawny owls) so is the most commonly seen owl, particularly while hunting small animals on marshlands. And if you don't see them, you are likely to hear the tawny owls' distinctive twit-twoo at dawn or dusk when they are noisiest. The sound is a mesmerising call and response between male and female as they search for a mate.

Of course, robins are the most famous bird of the Yule season – perhaps because they are easiest to spot due to their festive red feathers, which are more abundant in Winter, and their bold nature, seeking worms for breakfast in domestic gardens. Their song, used to mark their territory, is always surprisingly loud for such a small bird.

The pike is the largest freshwater predatory fish in the UK; they can be seen congregating in shallow water such as lakes and reservoirs in lowland areas to lay and fertilise their eggs. They are long, glowing green and missile-shaped – so you're unlikely to miss them thrashing around if they are about!

An eerie sight, frogs and toads hibernate at the bottom of ponds and other bodies of water thanks to the constant low temperatures that sustain the low metabolism needed to survive the Winter. On bright days you might see their shadowy outline in shallower waterways.

FORAGING FOLIAGE

As well as using meaningful and sentimental pieces to decorate mindfully, I love to forage greenery in abundance to bring festive colour, texture and scent into my home. This tradition goes back to the Celts who celebrated the festival of Yule at the Winter Solstice with evergreens to symbolise everlasting life. Foraging wasn't just for decorating but also a deeply spiritual affair, with certain plants such as mistletoe thought to ward off evil spirits of the night. Evergreens would be hung around doorways and windows, and each has its own distinct symbolism.

A large Yule log was brought into the house and kindled at dusk on the Winter Solstice. Once lit, by the remnants of the previous year's log, it was not allowed to go out by itself but had to be deliberately extinguished and part of the log left for the next year. In the Scottish Highlands the figure of Cailleach – a Celtic goddess associated with landscape and the weather – was sometimes carved into the log and the family would watch the figure – representing Winter and death – ceremonially burn before gathering with games and feasting long into the night. Our modern tradition of tucking into a chocolate log at Christmas evolved from the customary burning of the Yule log.

The best places to forage for the below 'ingredients' are woods, hedgerows, verges and even gardens. Before you begin, make sure you have the landowner's permission and forage sparingly from each area. Make sure you can identify what you are taking and be on the lookout for evergreens, branches, berries, seed heads and more. When you get home, make sure to give your foraged finds a shake (outside) to get rid of any beasties, then get decorating!

Florist's wire is your friend for making mantelpiece swags and table runners (see page 186) and sprigs of individual cuttings in recycled glass bottles add cheer dotted around the house. I usually update my Autumn Wreath (see page 134) with more evergreen clippings and add a festive coloured ribbon. A simple, seasonal update.

Holly
(*Ilex aquifolium*)

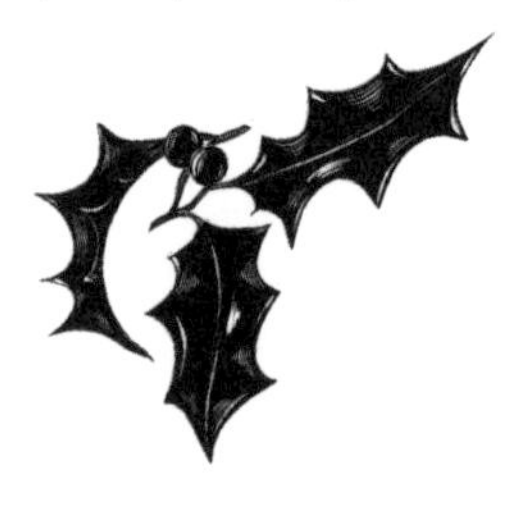

Holly is steeped in symbolism: our ancestors have been bringing holly inside during Winter for thousands of years: a reminder of hope, renewal and springtime to come during the darkest days and longest nights. The Celts considered holly a symbol of good luck, and in wreath form it represents friendship and faithful love. It was even thought to be unlucky to cut down a holly tree. This well-loved shrub is widely available in woodland, hedgerows and gardens. Get there early if you want to beat the birds to those festive red berries – and make sure you leave some for them.

Mistletoe
(*Viscum album*)

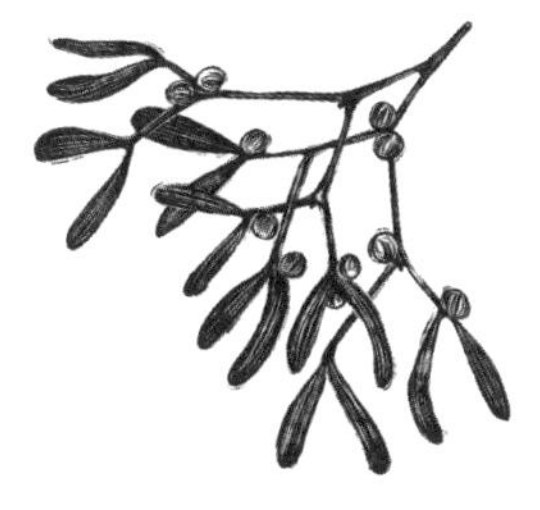

Mistletoe is a parasitic plant often found on apple and oak trees – where it was particularly revered by the Celts. Its forked branches hold pairs of evergreen leaves with pearl-like berries in Winter. In the past, the poisonous plant was hung above doors to prevent spirits from entering the home; however, thanks to the Celts and their association of mistletoe with fertility, the plant took on its modern meaning as a prompt for couples to kiss at Christmas. This association with Paganism and magic means that mistletoe is usually not included in church decorations – even to this day. Sadly, mistletoe doesn't grow abundantly in the wild in Scotland, so I usually get some from my local florist.

Ivy
(*Hedera helix*)

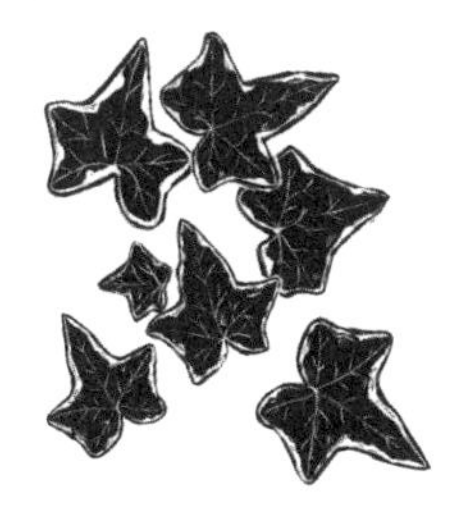

Ivy is a climber that grows almost anywhere: it is often found clinging to walls or trees with its small roots. In Celtic mythology it symbolises immortality, its spiral shape said to represent continuity and rebirth. Festive wreaths similarly represent the wheel of life, continuity and rebirth and are usually made with evergreens – ivy is ideal for this as it bends and twists with ease and retains moisture well. Contrary to popular belief, ivy doesn't harm trees but is a friend to many different species of wildlife; it is even thought to help preserve old buildings and keep them cool and damp-free.

Bracken
(*Pteridium aquilinum*)

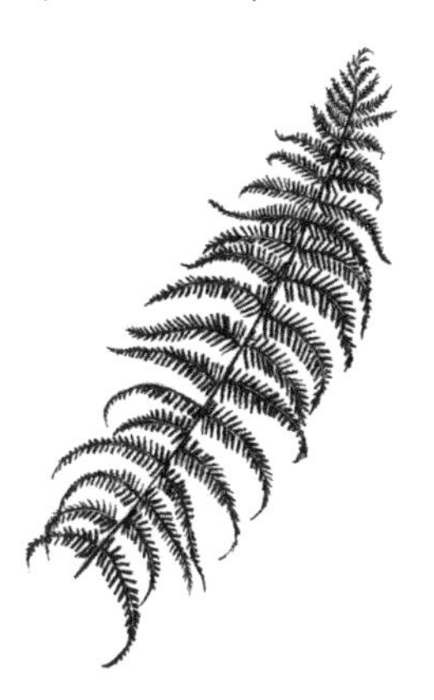

Bracken is a type of large, coarse, ancient fern. It is the most common species of fern in the UK and grows densely on hillsides, woods and moors. In the Winter it fades to shades of amber and burnt sienna as it withers and dies back. Bracken can be overpowering so is often cut back by councils and wildlife trusts. Myths and legends surround this plant too: it was thought to give perpetual youth and even invisibility. In Scottish folklore people thought the plant was in the shape of the devil's foot. Devilish or not, it adds beautiful texture and movement as well as earthy colour to displays and wreaths.

GREENERY GARLAND

Making a garland or shorter swag is a good way to create a lot with a little, and is quicker to make than a wreath if time isn't on your side. Not only do they save space, but they will bring the seasonal scent of fir into the home. They require minimal investment but offer instant Christmas spirit. Offcuts of branches can be sourced from local florists if you can't forage it, while some Christmas tree sellers even give away their offcuts for free. You can decorate a garland with whatever you have to hand – ribbons are particularly effective.

YOU WILL NEED

Several fir branches, or a mixture of fir, eucalyptus, larch, etc.
Florist's wire or twine
Scissors suitable for cutting wire or twine
Ribbon, bells and/or other decorations

Start by cutting all the foliage from your fir branches in small pieces. Make a small bundle with a few pieces and wrap the wire around them at the base; don't cut the wire yet.

Make another bundle and place it halfway over the first bundle so it overlaps, then attach with more wire.

Repeat, playing around with the foliage placement to provide depth and texture, keeping the wire attached underneath all the way along.

Keep going until you have either used up all your foliage or have achieved the length you want to create.

Position your garland where you want to display it, using more florist's wire to secure it.

Decorate your garland with ribbon offcuts, threaded through a small bell or bauble, if you like. Arrange in odd numbers for the best effect.

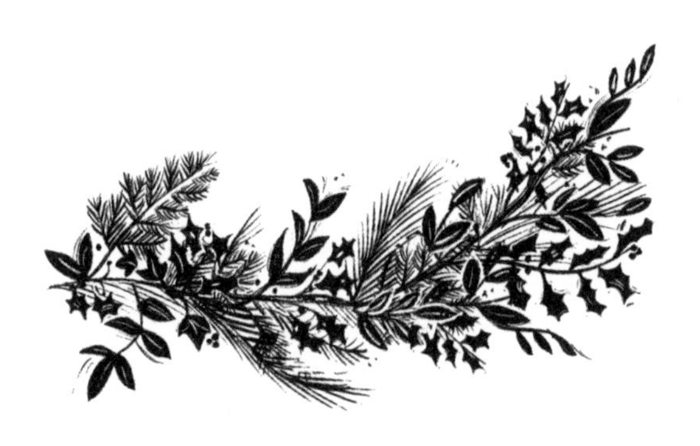

Ideas for your garland

- If you don't have much foliage, you could create a swag, which is shorter and hangs vertically – in this case, you would work from the bottom up. It should be lighter at the top and bulkier with more foliage at the bottom, so taper as you go by adding less foliage in each bundle, the higher up parts overlapping the bottom pieces. Hang from your front door instead of a wreath, decorating with a big ribbon tied in a bow at the top.
- Use a garland to decorate the banister of a staircase: make several shorter garlands and join them together in situ, letting each garland hang in an arc and securing to the banister with more wire, overlapping with the next arc, and so on.
- Use a shorter garland to decorate one end of your mantelpiece. Make sure the garland isn't hanging too close to the fire itself.
- You could add more foraging finds such as pine cones, dried honesty seed heads and dried orange slices inserted at intervals to give the arrangement depth and character.
- Keep your garland fresh by giving it a mist with water every other day and revive your garland by adding a little fresh foliage wired in with the older foliage that will begin to dry out.

Disposing of your foraged festive makes

- Most councils have a Christmas tree recycling service – be sure to look up your local area's rules online. Carefully remove all decorations, fairy lights and wire and simply add to the Christmas tree collection where trees will be shredded and composted.
- Or, if you have a stove, you could leave the wood to dry out completely, break up your branches and use them as kindling. Check the rules for what you can burn in your local area first.

TWIG STAR

This craft is best made with the straightest sticks you can find, so if you are making the other projects, set aside any helpful contenders. As long as you alternate weaving the twigs under and over one another, your star will be sturdier and hold itself together more readily. That said, these twig stars are meant to look rustic and will be all the more characterful for their slight wonkiness – nature isn't perfect, after all. You can make them in various sizes, but I'd start with bigger stars until you get the knack for it.

YOU WILL NEED

5 straight twigs (of roughly equal width)
Secateurs
Twine or string
Scissors

First, cut your twigs to the same length using the secateurs.

Take two sticks. Place the right hand stick on top of the left hand stick at a 30 degree angle and tie together with some twine or string: tie once, then loop around twice and tie again at the back to secure, then trim the twine or string. This is the top of the star.

At the opposite end of the left hand stick, place the third twig on top at a 30 degree angle, and tie together with twine in the same way to form the bottom left point of the star.

Place the fourth twig under the opposite end of the last stick you added (going horizontally underneath the top point of the star) to make the top right point of the star, tying it in securely to the third twig.

Add the fifth twig on top of the untied end of the fourth stick, passing it over the top left point of the star and under the bottom right point of the star. Tie into place to form the top left hand and bottom right hand points and complete the star.

Tip

You could tie several of these stars together into a garland, loop twine or string through to hang them on hooks, door handles or your front door, or scatter them over the table.

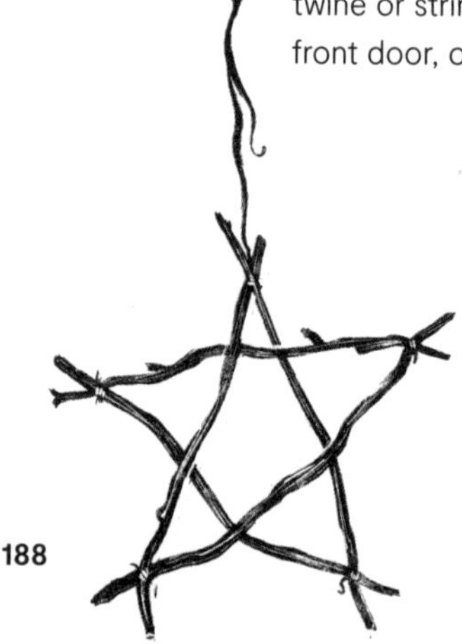

FESTIVE BRANCH

These days, many of us are living in small spaces and up several flights of stairs, particularly in the city. For the last few years, we haven't had room for a tree in our tiny tenement but still wanted to decorate with collected baubles and trinkets. Enter the festive branch! In the aftermath of the Winter's first storms, you will often find fallen branches and twigs that are sadly no longer of any use to the tree, which would only be chipped and composted once cleared by the local council. Ask the landowner's permission to remove them and they can be repurposed as a festive branch! Silver birch branches are particularly lovely for this craft as the pale bark will reflect the fairy lights. Measure the space where you want to hang your branches before you go foraging.

YOU WILL NEED

A couple of large branches
Pencil
Picture hooks or self-adhesive hooks
Hammer
Strong florist's wire
Battery-powered fairy lights
Decorations

Starting with the biggest, hold up the branches vertically in front of a blank wall and position how you want them. I try to follow the natural shapes of the tree and fill in gaps with smaller branches tucked behind.

As you're going to be adding decorations to the branch, you don't want it to fall over: you could place them in a pot with stones, but I always think it's safer to temporarily attach your branches to the wall. Holding the branches in position, identify a top, middle and bottom point on each branch where you can attach them with wire – and mark on the wall in pencil so you know where to put the hooks. Set the branches aside for now.

Attach the picture hooks at the marked positions on the wall, tapping them lightly into place with a hammer, or if you're using self-adhesive hooks, follow the instructions on the packet carefully.

Measure around 12cm wire for each hook, depending on the width of your branches. Loop the wire securely around the bottom of the picture hook several times, and then attach the other end to the branch, winding it around its girth several times.

Repeat until each branch is firmly tethered in place and feels stable.

Loop the fairy lights around the branches to decorate and hide the battery pack behind the branches at the back.

The tree will look beautiful as it is if you want. Otherwise, attach your decorations to the natural bends, twigs and nodules of the branches using their hooks, securing them with extra wire if needed.

Step back and admire your handiwork every so often to make sure your decorations are evenly spaced.

INDEX

ACKNOWLEDGEMENTS

My book wouldn't exist without these wonderful people. Thank you...

To my editor Kitty and the team for allowing me so much creative input and being so flexible around my day job; the evening meetings and holiday deadlines helped me keep the plates spinning!

To my agent Megan. Signing my contract with Bergstrom Studio on International Women's Day was a pinch-me moment. Thank you for rebuilding my confidence and teaching me to value what I have to offer.

To designer Lucy and illustrator Holly for bringing the book to life visually. Lucy, you made a book packed with projects welcoming and readable and Holly, your illustrations are so beautiful – it's like you can see inside my brain!

To the teachers who believed in me. To the supportive colleagues and young people, past and present, who inspire me every day. You know who you are.

To Ronnie and Sarah, you truly changed my life.

To friends and family who helped me test the recipes and crafts in these pages. To my readers and followers over the years – I appreciate every single one of you. To the writers who have supported me: Beth Kempton, Laura Pashby, Lucy Brazier, Jess Elliott Dennison and others.

To Mum, for instilling a love of making. I learnt so much watching you and Gran. To Dad, for your support and sampling much marmalade over the years! To Jamie, for the many adventures along the Avenue, past and present, and pavlova experiment encouragement.

To Gran and Granda, we miss you every single day.

To Al, I couldn't have done any of it without you. Thank you for seeing all of me. I love you so much.

Rosie Steer embraced slow living and found solace in the ancient nature-centric traditions of the Celtic Wheel of the Year after suffering with her mental health. She set up her blog and platform on Instagram, @everythinglooksrosie, as a place to track small moments of joy through the seasons and fostered a loyal following in the process. She lives and works in Edinburgh.

BLOOMSBURY PUBLISHING
Bloomsbury Publishing Plc
50 Bedford Square, London, WC1B 3DP, UK
29 Earlsfort Terrace, Dublin 2, Ireland

BLOOMSBURY, BLOOMSBURY PUBLISHING and the Diana logo are trademarks of Bloomsbury Publishing Plc

First published in Great Britain 2023

A catalogue record for this book is available from the British Library

Library of Congress Cataloguing-in-Publication data has been applied for

ISBN: HB: 978-1-5266-6272-9; eBook: 978-1-5266-6273-6

10 9 8 7 6 5 4 3 2

Copy editor: Claire Rogers
Designer: Studio Polka
Illustrator: Holly Ovenden

Printed and bound in Slovenia by DZS Grafik.

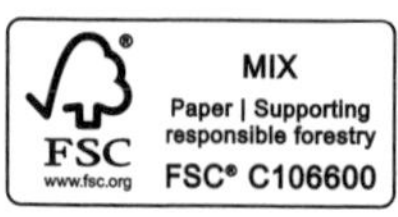

To find out more about our authors and books visit www.bloomsbury.com and sign up for our newsletters